Fertility Preservation - Theory and Practice Experience

Edited by Wei Wu and Hongshan Ge

Published in London, United Kingdom

Fertility Preservation - Theory and Practice Experience
http://dx.doi.org/10.5772/intechopen.1005719
Edited by Wei Wu and Hongshan Ge

Contributors
Chenglu Wang, Constantina Claudia Mateoiu, Feng-xia Liu, Georgi Stamenov, Giulia Orlandi, Ka-li Huang, Kameliya Kostadinova, Leixiang Yang, Min Zheng, Songlin Zhang, Tanya Timeva, Xiaohua Tang, Xiaopan Chen, Zhong Lin

First published in London, United Kingdom, 2026 by IntechOpen
IntechOpen is the global imprint of INTECHOPEN LIMITED, registered in England and Wales, registration number: 11086078, 167-169 Great Portland Street, London, W1W 5PF, United Kingdom

For EU product safety concerns: IN TECH d.o.o., Prolaz Marije Krucifikse Kozulić 3, 51000 Rijeka, Croatia, info@intechopen.com or visit our website at intechopen.com.

British Library Cataloguing-in-Publication Data
A catalogue record for this book is available from the British Library

Fertility Preservation - Theory and Practice Experience
Edited by Wei Wu and Hongshan Ge
p. cm.

This title is part of the Obstetrics and Gynecology Book Series, Volume 15
Topic: Reproductive and Gynecologic Health
Series Editor: Zouhair O. Amarin
Topic Editor: Courtney Marsh

Print ISBN 978-1-83634-983-9
Online ISBN 978-1-83634-982-2
eBook (PDF) ISBN 978-1-83634-984-6
ISSN 3049-706X

If disposing of this product, please recycle the paper responsibly.

IntechOpen Book Series

Obstetrics and Gynecology

Volume 15

Aims and Scope of the Series

Obstetrics and Gynecology field typically covers several subspecialties that include maternal-fetal medicine, gynecologic oncology, reproductive endocrinology and subfertility, urogynecology and female pelvic reconstructive surgery, critical care medicine, complex family planning, pediatric and adolescent gynecology, menopausal and geriatric gynecology, and minimally invasive gynecologic surgery.
Apart from being diverse, obstetrics and gynecology is a challenging and demanding specialty. It combines medical and surgical skills.
The sequence of books in this series will have certain characteristics in common that will be recognized as part of the same informative multi-volume book programme.

Meet the Series Editor

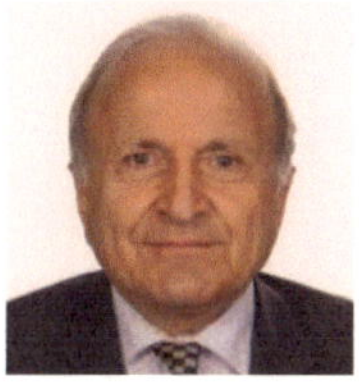

Zouhair Amarin is a Professor of Obstetrics and Gynaecology at the Jordan University of Science and Technology. He was previously a lecturer at the University of Glasgow, Scotland, a senior lecturer at the University of Nottingham, England, and the dean of the Faculty of Medicine at Mutah University, Jordan. Professor Amarin is a fellow of the Royal College of Obstetricians and Gynaecologists, and the Faculty of Public Health, London. He holds master's degrees in medical science and medical education. He is a pioneer in IVF and was the first in the world to develop microsurgical epididymis sperm aspiration for clinical use. He also discovered a surgical procedure for critical ovarian hyperstimulation syndrome. Professor Amarin has edited books, authored book chapters, and published more than 130 papers. He is the recipient of eight awards.

Meet the Volume Editors

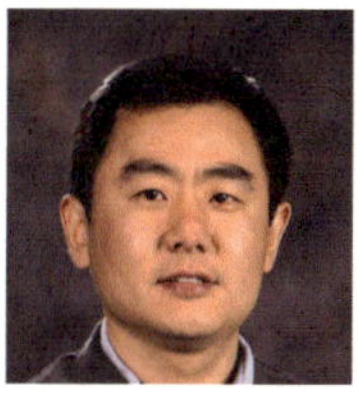

Dr. Wei Wu serves as Deputy Dean of the School of International Education, Deputy Director of the Department of International Cooperation and Exchange, and Professor of the Department of Toxicology at Nanjing Medical University, China. He was a guest researcher at the National Institute of Environmental Health Sciences (NIEHS) between 2017 and 2018. He is the PI of the State Key Laboratory of Reproductive Medicine and Offspring Health, and the Key Laboratory of Modern Toxicology of the Ministry of Education. He is a member of several national and international societies in the fields of human reproduction and toxicology, and has received awards from many of these societies for the originality and quality of his projects. He has a wide range of teaching and consulting experience, including in toxicology. His research interests include the application of new media technology in teaching, epigenetic mechanisms underlying the transgenerational effects of male infertility induced by endocrine-disrupting chemicals and environmental exposure, and genetic and epigenetic risk factors for male infertility and abnormal fetal growth. Prof. Wu has published 100+ papers in peer-reviewed journals, including Environmental Pollution, EBioMedicine, Environment International, Environmental Health, Clinical Epigenetics, Toxicological Sciences, Human Reproduction, and Molecular Human Reproduction. He has edited 9 books, collaborated on 10 books and 19 patents, and served on the organizing committees of 3 international conferences. Prof. Wu serves as the Editor-in-Chief of the International Journal of Sexual Health and Reproductive Health Care, Research International Journal of Endocrinology and Diabetes, Executive Editor of Annals of Molecular and Genetic Medicine, Associate Editor of the JSM Invitro Fertilization, and editor of many other journals, including Scientific Reports and Experimental and Therapeutic Medicine.

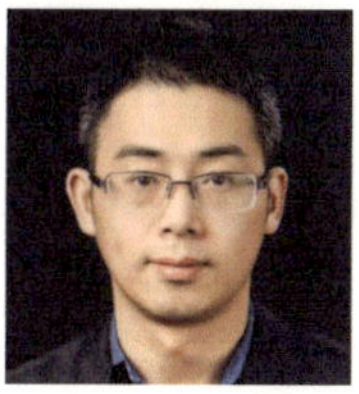

Dr. Hongshan Ge, MD, Professor, currently directs the Obstetrics and Gynecology and Reproductive Center at Taizhou People's Hospital, in association with Nanjing Medical University. Prior to his current role, he served as Deputy Director in the Department of Obstetrics and Gynecology at both the Second Clinical College and the Second Affiliated Hospital of Wenzhou Medical University. Dr. Ge possesses 22 years of experience in reproductive medicine, specializing in the clinical application of Assisted Reproductive Technologies (ART) and the comprehensive management of female infertility. He has successfully managed over 10,000 ART cycles, including conventional IVF/ICSI treatments, IVM, and oocyte cryopreservation. Dr. Ge's research focuses on the pathophysiology of polycystic ovary syndrome (PCOS) and premature ovarian insufficiency (POI), and on the role of mitochondrial function in gamete and embryonic development. He has published over 80 peer-reviewed articles and contributed to a scholarly monograph, thereby significantly advancing the field's knowledge base and clinical practices in reproductive health.

Contents

Preface

This Edited Volume, *Fertility Preservation – Theory and Practice Experience*, is a collection of reviewed and relevant research chapters on developments in the field of gynecology. The book includes scholarly contributions from various authors and is edited by experts in this field. Each contribution comes as a separate chapter complete in itself but directly related to the book's topics and objectives.

The book includes the following chapters:

1. Obstetric Outcome of Pregnancy from AID

2. Endometrial Assessment to Ensure Successful Implantation

3. The Role of Gynaecological Pathology in Fertility Preservation: Theory and Practical Experience

4. Expanding the Role of BNIP3 in Autophagy: Hypoxia-Induced Primordial Follicle Loss and Perspectives for Ischemia-Reperfusion Injury in Ovarian Tissue Transplantation

5. Fertility Preservation in Hematological Malignancies: A Growing Imperative

6. Epigenetic Stability and Genomic Integrity in Fertility Preservation: Insights from Genetic and Reproductive Technologies

IntechOpen

Chapter 1

Obstetric Outcome of Pregnancy from AID

Giulia Orlandi

Abstract

This chapter describes the obstetric outcomes of pregnancies from PMA-heterologous. An effective preconception assessment of patients with indication for heterologous PMA with oocyte donation is necessary through the evaluation of comorbidities, cardio-metabolic, and thrombophilia markers of obstetric risk. This is useful to try to improve the obstetric outcome of this group of pregnancies at risk of major obstetric complications and neonatal complications. Investigating and correcting any co-pathologies before implanting the embryos in the uterus helps to reduce the risk of complications. All PMA centers should proceed to carry out this check before performing assisted fertilization in order to reduce negative obstetric outcomes and any secondary neonatal complications.

Keywords: pregnancy rate, obstetrics complications, immunological aspects, placenta, AID

1. Introduction

Considering the great success rate of pregnancies from oocyte donation, it is plausible to assume that the majority of women who undergo this procedure are able to successfully finish their pregnancies. An analysis of 500 consecutive cycles of oocyte donation, going back to the early 1990s, showed that over half the recipients achieved a pregnancy at the third embryo transfer, irrespective of age or the pathology that represented the indication for PMA-E (**Figure 1**) [1].

Moment, with public birth rates of 50–60% per embryo transfer, it is reasonable to assume that success can be achieved in 75–90% of cases who have experienced multiple attempts at heterologous fertilization [2]. Still, this success is accompanied by the observation of multitudinous obstetric complications that may arise during gestation.

2. Obstetric complications

Donated egg pregnancies are linked to negative outcomes for both the mother and newborn. Various aspects that differentiate these pregnancies from those achieved through natural conception and standard IVF methods might clarify this link:

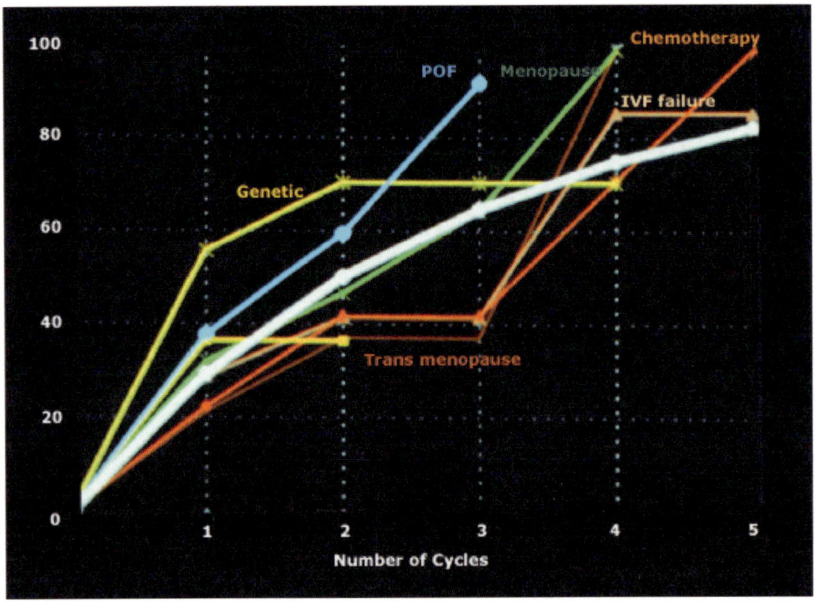

Figure 1.
Success rates after oocyte donation [1].

- the method itself, meaning the ovarian stimulation treatment which affects the endometrial lining, the unique implantation resulting from embryo transfer, and the fact that the initial development of the trophoblast takes place outside the uterus;
- the age of the mother, which is often older;
- the higher occurrence of multiple pregnancies.

Following the initial experience of pregnancy through heterologous fertilization with egg donation, research aimed at evaluating obstetric results has revealed a higher rate of preeclampsia and gestational hypertension [3, 4]. Additional studies indicate a greater likelihood of low birth weight, premature births, and cesarean deliveries in pregnancies from egg donation when compared to those achieved via traditional fertilization methods [5, 6]. Gestational hypertensive conditions, such as chronic hypertension, gestational hypertension, preeclampsia/eclampsia, and HELLP syndrome, contribute significantly to maternal morbidity and mortality around the globe. These conditions are also linked to preterm births and babies with low birth weights. Specifically, in highly developed countries, these health issues are responsible for 16 percent of maternal mortality cases [7].

Four meta-analyses have been released that explore obstetric complications among egg donor patients. The analysis conducted by Pecks et al. [8] examines the rates of hypertensive disorders and preeclampsia across heterologous, homologous, and spontaneous pregnancies: it reports a notable increase in the risk of hypertensive disorders in egg donor pregnancies compared to homologous (AOR 2.57) and spontaneous pregnancies (AOR 6.60). However, two of the five studies that compared egg donors to spontaneous conceptions did not account for the occurrence of multiple pregnancies, which may help explain the higher risk observed in egg donors.

Masoudian and his team found that the likelihood of developing preeclampsia is four times higher in pregnancies from egg donors than in those that occur naturally (Adjusted Odds Ratio 4.34), without taking multiple gestations into account. Additionally, they reported an adjusted odds ratio of 2.24 when comparing singleton pregnancies from egg donation with those from primary medical-assisted (PMA-O) sources [9]. A recent literature review by Storgaard and colleagues in 2016 reaffirmed these findings, indicating that singleton pregnancies resulting from heterologous methods have double the risk of preeclampsia (adjusted odds ratio 2.11) compared to homologous pregnancies and tripled for multiple gestations (adjusted odds ratio 3.31), even after considering the age of the mothers. In a study conducted in Sweden, it was discovered that gestational hypertension, preeclampsia, and other pregnancy-related complications are more frequent in assisted reproductive technology using egg donors (ART-E) than in those using own eggs (ART-O), even among young recipients without chronic health issues [10]. It is suggested that the variations in placentation associated with hypertensive complications may be a response from the mother's immune system to a genetically different fetus [8, 11, 12]. This hypothesis is supported by histological and immunohistochemical research that shows a higher occurrence of placental abnormalities, including villitis, chronic deciduitis, chronic villositis, placental infarction, and ischemic changes in the maternal–fetal boundary [13, 14].

There are various other obstetric issues that can arise in pregnancies resulting from egg donation, with postpartum hemorrhage being particularly significant from a clinical perspective. The rate of this complication in singleton pregnancies from PMA-E ranges from 4.2 to 17.3%, while in IVF pregnancies, it varies from 0 to 9.3%. The risk is raised in single pregnancies (adjusted odds ratio 2. 4) and is notably higher in twin pregnancies (adjusted odds ratio 4.91) [15].

Regarding the incidence of gestational diabetes, seven different studies were performed, showing a range of 0–13% in singleton pregnancies from PMA-E and between 1 and 23.3% in IVF pregnancies, compared to only 1.1% in naturally conceived pregnancies according to Nejdet et al. [5]. There has been no study indicating a significant difference in gestational diabetes rates among the different types of pregnancies. Four of the studies provided information on gestational diabetes in multiple gestations: the incidence ranged from 0–31% in egg donation cases and from 1.7–8% in IVF pregnancies. In two of these studies, the likelihood of developing gestational diabetes was notably higher in heterologous pregnancies.

From a neonatal viewpoint, a meta-analysis conducted in 2015 indicated a notable rise in the chances of both low birth weight and preterm births [16]. This finding aligns with data collected from a group of women from Sweden and Denmark, who reported an adjusted odds ratio of 1.53 for low birth weight and 1.75 for preterm birth when contrasting pregnancies from egg donors with traditional pregnancies. This situation can be partly attributed to the growing number of elective cesarean deliveries occurring before the 40th week of pregnancy. The prevalence of cesarean sections is actually more than double in pregnancies involving preterm maternal age compared to any other pregnancy type, as these are primarily planned surgical procedures. The research conducted by Malchau and colleagues is notable for exclusively presenting the figures for both elective and emergency cesarean sections, revealing roughly equivalent rates.

Given that pregnancies from egg donations occur two to three times more than standard IVF pregnancies, we would expect a similarly significant rise in the occurrence of small for gestational age infants. According to the findings reported by

Lashley and associates, there were no instances of small for gestational age in the nine heterologous pregnancies impacted by preeclampsia, while 30% of small for gestational age infants were found in those conceived by mothers with preeclampsia undergoing assisted reproductive technology, leading to a statistically meaningful difference. It is surprising that hypertensive disorders such as preeclampsia have a lower impact on pregnancy from egg donation compared to singleton IVF pregnancies, but this concept requires further research on the underlying pathophysiological mechanism.

The utilization of freezing techniques is probably associated with higher birth weight, and this technique could influence the outcome; however, it is not clear in the studies performed, whether the oocytes or embryos utilized were frozen [5]. The development of the uterus also plays an important role, in fact women of advanced maternal age who have conceived spontaneously at a young age, bring advantages in terms of growth to the fetus [12, 17], compared to women with other types of reproductive pathologies, who are therefore nulliparous at the time of heterologous fertilization. Egg donor pregnancies two to three times more than traditional IVF pregnancies, we would expect the number of SGAs to increase equally significantly. However, this is not demonstrated in the most recent meta-analysis and the number of SGA infants has not been taken into account in obstetric outcomes in other published reviews. In the study by Lashley et al., no cases of SGA were found in the nine heterologous pregnancies complicated by preeclampsia, compared to 30% of SGA conceived by preeclamptic mothers undergoing ART, resulting in a statistically significant difference [18].

It is surprising that hypertensive disorders such as preeclampsia have a lower impact on pregnancy from egg donation compared to singleton IVF pregnancies, but this concept requires further research on the underlying pathophysiological mechanism. The use of freezing techniques is probably associated with higher birth weight, and this technique could influence the outcome, but it is not clear in the studies performed, whether the oocytes or embryos used were frozen [5]. The development of the uterus also plays an important role, in fact women of advanced maternal age who have conceived spontaneously at a young age bring benefits in terms of growth to the fetus, compared to women with other types of reproductive pathologies, who are therefore nulliparous at the time of heterologous fertilization.

3. Immunological aspects in pregnancy from PMA-heterologous

Spontaneous pregnancy is an immunological paradox itself. The fetus receives genetic material from both the mother and father, but the mother's immune system does not reject it during the entire course of the pregnancy.

Particular immune mechanisms operate in natural pregnancies that help to clarify how mothers tolerate their developing fetus.

Because fetal tissue directly interacts with maternal blood, it is vulnerable to attacks from the mother's innate and adaptive immune responses, which could result in the death of the fetus.

This vulnerability led to the evolution of a maternal–fetal interface that facilitates immune tolerance.

The fundamental process involves the "down-regulation" of the maternal immune response, preventing it from attacking the semi-allogeneic fetus, which enables the embryo to implant and grow.

It is widely accepted that a successful pregnancy hinges on the balance of different elements of maternal immunity and the actions of T helper 2 lymphocytes involved in cell-mediated immunity.

Within the maternal–fetal interface, identifying fetal antigens, delivered by trophoblast or fetal cells in the maternal bloodstream, is crucial for activating immune mechanisms.

Indeed, it appears that alongside T lymphocytes in this area, there exist additional cells that modulate the activity of T lymphocytes.

It is these cells that facilitate the previously mentioned down-regulation process.

For PMA-E pregnancies, more non-maternal antigens are present than in a fetus stemming from spontaneous conception. Considering the five most prevalent HLA antigens, specifically HLA-A, -B, -C, -DR, and –DQ, the utmost number of mismatches that will appear in a spontaneous pregnancy is 5. In a PMA-E pregnancy, the count for the same HLA will be 10 (**Figure 2**).

In addition, blood samples from women undergoing ART also show a higher percentage of γintracellular interferon (Th1), interleukin-4, and CD4+ Th2 lymphocytes, compared to the percentage found in blood samples from women who have undertaken a spontaneous pregnancy [19]. Th1 and Th2 hyperactivation, induced by the allogeneic fetus, is a specific characteristic of pregnancy from oocyte donation.

This indicates that the Th2-driven process promotes the success of pregnancies achieved through assisted reproductive techniques, even when the conceived product is entirely foreign. The research conducted by Chernyshov and colleagues in 2008, which examined immune cells taken from maternal blood samples, led to the finding that the active immune processes occur at the maternal–fetal interface. Thus, it was proposed that the related effects are primarily seen in this area. A recent study has identified a notable link between HLA mismatches and the levels of activated CD4+ and CD25 T cells present in the decidua during normal pregnancies [20]. Additionally, in natural pregnancies, researchers have explored the connection between the

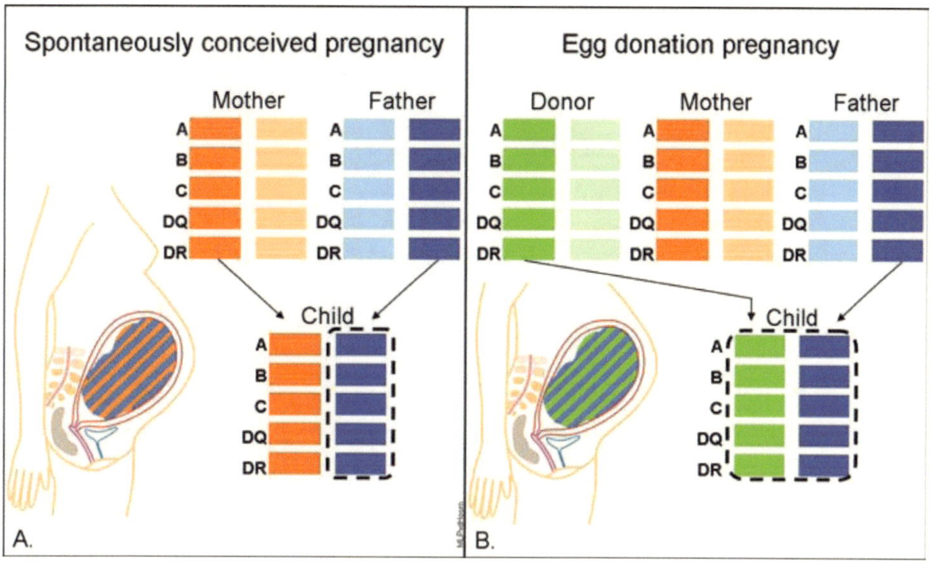

Figure 2.
Interaction of the most common HLA antigens in a spontaneous pregnancy and in a pregnancy from egg donation [14].

quantity of mismatched amino acid triplets (HLA epitopes) between the mother and the fetus and the mother's production of antibodies against paternal antigens that the fetus has inherited. A significant association has been observed between the number of mismatches in triplets and the rate of women who produce HLA antibodies. When there are no matching amino acid triplets between the mother and the fetus, antibodies will not be generated, even if there are one or more mismatches in HLA antigens. It is still to be determined whether the total number of mismatches in HLA or in epitopes is more crucial for achieving fetal tolerance. In any scenario, pregnancies from donor eggs exhibit a higher count of both HLA antigens and epitopes compared to pregnancies resulting from natural conception (**Figure 3**).

Therefore, the percentage of women who produce antibodies is also higher, which can lead to implications during the clinical phase. Hence, we can conclude that the immune system plays an essential role in the processes related to pregnancies achieved through egg donation. Unfortunately, we do not have information about the long-term impacts that might arise throughout the life of the recipient woman, considering her previous exposure to foreign antigens and cells. It is therefore important to explore the reasons that led the recipient to pursue the PMA-E method. For example, regarding primary ovarian failure, it is widely accepted that an autoimmune process is involved in the onset of the condition. It is likely that this autoimmunity contributes to the differences in the immune response observed between pregnancies resulting from PMA-E and those achieved through natural conception.

The maternal–fetal interface of the placenta from egg donation shows several and notable differences compared to that of a pregnancy achieved from spontaneous conception. Indeed, a greater frequency of histological lesions attributable to villitis of unknown etiology, chronic deciduitis, chronic massive intervillositis, and ischemic-type alterations has been documented, meaning all those conditions also more often observed in pregnant women affected by preeclampsia (**Figure 4**) [13, 21].

Deciduitis, which develops in these placentas, is noted for its intensity and the significant fibrin build-up found on the basal plate. In this same area, there is a prominent presence of lymphocytes, especially CD4+ Th lymphocytes and CD56+ NK lymphocytes. Additionally, in the basal plate, the extra villous trophoblast, originating from the fetus, interacts with and penetrates the maternal tissues. The cells of the

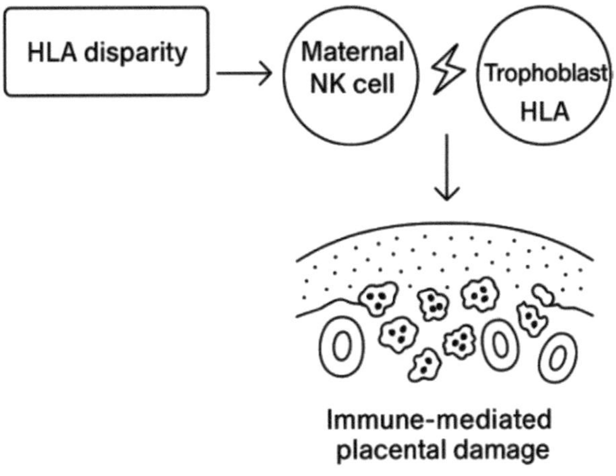

Figure 3.
HLA disparity triggers immune-mediated placental damage.

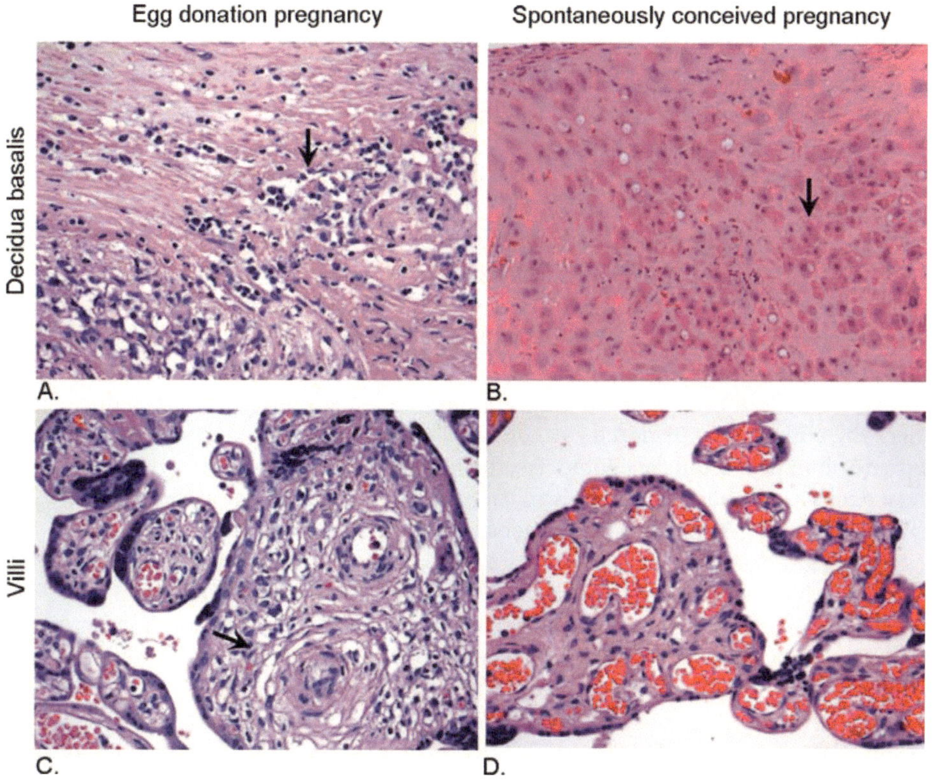

Figure 4.
Microscopic images of a placenta from egg donation and from spontaneous pregnancy. (A) Basal decidua of a placenta from egg donation with deciduitis illustrated by monocytic infiltration. (B) Normal basal decidua in a placenta from spontaneous pregnancy and normal decidual cells. (C) Villi in a placenta from egg donation. A rich lymphocytic infiltrate is present in the stroma. (D) Villi in a placenta from spontaneous pregnancy (From the Hoorn, 2010).

extra villous trophoblast lack the typical HLA-A and HLA-B molecules, which inhibits engagement with cytotoxic T cells. Nonetheless, they display a distinct mix of HLA antigens (HLA-C, along with the non-conventional HLA-E and HLA-G) that interact with KIR receptors found on uterine natural killer (uNK) cells [22–25], although HLA-C may also act as a target for CD8+ T cells [20].

Therefore, the finding of dense fibrin deposits and a high lymphocytic infiltration in the basal plate suggests an immune-mediated response that is more present in placentas of pregnancies obtained by heterologous fertilization. Placental damage may be due to a type of "graft-versus-host reaction disease" and/or a type of organ rejection [13].

More studies are required to verify if mismatches in HLA-C epitopes hinder the invasion of trophoblasts [26].

4. Discussion

Pregnancies resulting from egg donation (OD) are becoming more prevalent, as is the scientific field's interest in the impact of these procedures on maternal–fetal results.

The number of pregnancies resulting from egg donation is set to rise, particularly in women over 40. There are many causes for this trend, one of the most important being the shift in the concept of motherhood. Women tend to delay motherhood without regarding it a priority until they reach an advanced age. The medical community must be well informed of this social behavior and must be prepared to manage these "older pregnancies".

The obstetric complications in pregnancies resulting from assisted reproduction techniques are well documented; however, until recently the hazards associated with egg donation pregnancies were not known.

Egg donation has now been demonstrated to be an independent risk factor for hypertensive disease in pregnancy, postpartum hemorrhage, and increased risk of cesarean section.

The theory of immunological mal-adaptation of pregnancies from egg donation, where the embryo is considered as a totally allogeneic graft for the woman, is well known and in part totally accepted. In addition to this immunological theory, it seems that a decisive role has also been given to the hormonal preparation that precedes embryo transfer. We know that estrogens have an essential role in the placenta, promoting angiogenesis and the development of the vascularization of the placental villi [27]. It has recently been shown that the hyperestrogenic environment generated during ovarian stimulation can create a suboptimal environment that damages implantation by suppressing trophoblastic remodeling of the uterine spiral arteries, which leads to placental dysfunction and low birth weight [28].

Successful placentation and embryonic/fetal growth depend on optimal vascularization of the villous portion of the placenta [27]. It is plausible, in fact, that hormone administration at the beginning of pregnancy can modify the normal endocrine environment and interfere with early placentation events.

Regulatory T cells (Tregs) and uterine natural killer (uNK) cells are crucial for the success of pregnancy, where Tregs help establish tolerance for the fetus, and uNK cells assist with the development of the placenta. Changes in these cell types [29], whether through imbalances or loss of function, have been associated with negative pregnancy results such as repeated miscarriages, preeclampsia, and early delivery.

Some research suggests a decline in Treg counts, while other studies propose that it may be the dysfunction of Tregs rather than their numbers that poses a problem. Specifically, in cases of premature birth, research indicates a rise in pro-inflammatory cytokines, with certain types of Tregs, like memory Tregs, being more prevalent. The literature often discusses Tregs, suggesting that their reduced numbers or functionality could serve as a critical indicator of early labor. The differences in Treg research findings reflect the intricate nature of the immune environment in spontaneous preterm birth (sPTB), emphasizing the necessity for uniform research efforts to fully grasp the role of Tregs across various sPTB types.

Finally, we know that the coexistence of traditional cardiovascular risk factors in the preconceptionally period, often found in egg donor patients in relation to advanced maternal age, such as insulin resistance, obesity, systemic inflammation, preexisting hypertension, diabetes, and kidney disease, can influence the onset of preeclampsia.

To start with, maternal obesity is a significant public health concern that is increasingly becoming more serious. This condition presents specific risks for both the mother and the fetus throughout the entire pregnancy. Notable among these are pregnancy-related hypertension, venous thromboembolism, miscarriage, the need for labor induction, cesarean delivery, infections, and complications related to surgical wounds. Women with obesity or severe obesity are more likely to develop gestational diabetes, as excess weight impairs insulin function and increases the likelihood of negative effects on metabolism and cardiovascular health. Hyperinsulinism associated with obesity is considered a primary factor contributing to the higher incidence of hypertension in pregnant women dealing with obesity [30], leading to left ventricular hypertrophy due to heightened pre- and afterload, which can diminish contraction volume and overall heart performance. This situation results in ongoing hypoxia, hypercapnia, and pulmonary hypertension, which significantly elevate risks of illness and mortality for mothers, as indicated by findings from the Confidential Enquiry into Maternal and Child Health (CEMACH), which noted that 27% of maternal fatalities between 2013 and 2015 were in women with obesity (BMI > 30) [31].

In addressing chronic illnesses like diabetes, it is crucial to manage blood sugar levels effectively before conception (with HbA1c of 40), and being of advanced age (>45 years) necessitates establishing a collaborative care approach involving an obstetrician–gynecologist to evaluate these individuals.

It is essential for these women to receive thorough guidance on the increased risks associated with pregnancies from egg donation, along with a preconception health assessment to identify any existing conditions such as hypertension and diabetes before commencing fertility treatment. This conversation should also cover recommendations regarding elective single embryo transfer, as multiple births elevate the risk of complications, particularly preterm delivery and gestational diabetes. Moreover, they should have diligent oversight throughout the prenatal phase by a multidisciplinary team within a level III birthing facility.

Future studies should focus on effective methods to mitigate risks during egg donation pregnancies for both mothers and babies in the prenatal stage, during delivery, and in the postnatal period.

Many women who visit our preconception clinic do not fully understand the potential obstetric hazards they might encounter when pursuing a pregnancy through egg donation. Therefore, it is vital to offer preconception counseling to couples to help them comprehend the journey ahead. Conversely, couples seeking fertility treatments abroad often lack proper information and remain overly optimistic, not recognizing the full scope of risks due to inadequate education on the topic.

Private clinics, particularly those located overseas, often adopt an overly aggressive approach toward older patients, failing to take into account that the age-related restrictions set by Italian law 40 differ significantly from those in other European countries where egg donation practices are employed.

There are additional dangers related to ART procedures in older women who have undergone treatments outside the country, such as unrecognized mental and physical health conditions, since many clinics lack access to medical records, resulting in insufficient or fragmented medical histories of ongoing health issues. Some women might not fully understand the potential ramifications or may be determined to pursue pregnancy despite the associated risks.

It is crucial for society to become more conscious of the dangers involved and to foster greater dialog about reproductive matters linked to higher maternal age. Cryopreservation of eggs for later use is recommended as a potential solution to prevent DO in specific circumstances.

The necessity for future medical interventions is also a social and healthcare concern that requires increased attention to ensure that strategies are established to safeguard both the health of the woman and the developing child in the long and short term.

We cannot act on some adverse obstetric outcomes that are independent of the PMA-E technique, such as postpartum hemorrhage, cesarean section, and preeclampsia. What we can do is correct the metabolic risk by modifying the pre-pregnancy BMI and pre-conceptional glycemic values.

Author details

Giulia Orlandi
Dottoressa Giulia Orlandi, Azienda USL Toscana Centro, Ospedale San Jacopo Pistoia, Dipartimento Materno-Infantile, Italy

*Address all correspondence to: dottoressa.orlandi@gmail.com

References

[1] Paulson RJ, Hatch IE, Lobo RA, Sauer MV. Cumulative conception and live birth rates after oocyte donation: Implications regarding endometrial receptivity. Human Reproduction. 1997;**12**:835

[2] Ameratunga D, Weston G, Osianlis T, et al. In vitro fertilisation (IVF) with donor eggs in post-menopausal women: Are there differences in pregnancy outcomes in women with premature ovarian failure (POF) compared with women with physiological age-related menopause? Journal of Assisted Reproduction and Genetics. 2009;**26**:511

[3] Saito S, Sakai M. Th1/Th2 balance in preeclampsia. Journal of Reproductive Immunology. 2003;**59**:161-173

[4] Soderstrom-Anttila V, Tiitinen A, Foudila T, Hovatta O. Obstetric and perinatal outcome after oocyte donation: Comparison with in-vitro fertilization pregnancies. Human Reproduction. 1998;**13**:483-490

[5] Nejdet S, Bergh C, Kallén K, Wennerholm U, Thurin-Kjellberg A. High risks of maternal and perinatal complications in singletons born after oocyte donation. Acta Obstetricia et Gynecologica Scandinavica. 2016;**95**:879-886

[6] Soderstrom-Anttila V. Pregnancy and child outcome after oocyte donation. Human Reproduction Update. 2001;7:28-32

[7] Steegers EA, Von Dadelszen P, Duvekot JJ, Pijnenborg R. Preeclampsia. Lancet. 2010;**376**:631-644

[8] Pecks U, Maass N, Neulen J. Oocyte donation: A risk factor for pregnancy-induced hypertension: A meta-analysis and case series. Deutsches Ärzteblatt International. 2011;**108**(3):23-31

[9] Masoudian P, Nasr A, de Nanassy J, Fung-Kee-Fung K, Bainbridge SA, El Demellawy D. Oocyte donation pregnancies and the risk of preeclampsia or gestational hypertension: A systematic review and metaanalysis. American Journal of Obstetrics and Gynecology. 2016;**214**:328-339

[10] Elenis E et al. Adverse obstetric outcomes in pregnancies resulting from oocyte donation: A retrospective cohort case study in Sweden. BMC Pregnancy and Childbirth. 2015;**15**:247

[11] Levron Y, Dviri M, Segol I, Yerushalmi GM, Hourvitz A, Orvieto R, et al. The 'immunologic theory' of preeclampsia revisited: A lesson from donor oocyte gestations. American Journal of Obstetrics and Gynecology. 2014;**211**:383-385

[12] Younis JS, Laufer N. Oocyte donation is an independent risk factor for pregnancy complications: The implications for women of advanced age. Journal of Women's Health (Larchmont). Feb 2015;**24**(2):127-130. DOI: 10.1089/jwh.2014.4999. Epub 2015 Feb 3

[13] Gundogan F, Bianchi DW, Scherjon SA, Roberts DJ. Placental pathology in egg donor pregnancies. Fertility and Sterility. 2009;**93**:397-404

[14] Van Der Hoorn ML, Lashley EE, Bianchi DW, Claas FH, Schonkeren CM, Scherjon SA. Clinical and immunologic aspects of egg donation pregnancies: A systematic review. Human Reproduction Update. 2010;**16**:704-712

[15] Storgaard M, Loft A, Bergh C, Wennerholm UB, Soderstrom-Anttila V, Romundstad LB, et al. Obstetric and neonatal complications in pregnancies conceived after oocyte donation: A systematic review and meta-analysis. BJOG. 2017;**124**:561-572

[16] Adams DH, Clark RA, Davies MJ, de Lacey S. A meta-analysis of neonatal health outcomes from oocyte donation. Journal of Developmental Origins of Health and Disease. 2015;7:1-16

[17] Waldenström U, Cnattingius S, Vixner L, Norman M. Advanced maternal age increases the risk of very preterm birth, irrespective of parity: A population-based register study. BJOG. 2016

[18] Lashley LE, Buurma A, Swings GM, Eikmans M, Anholts JD, Bakker JA, et al. Preeclampsia in autologous and oocyte donation pregnancy: Is there a different pathophysiology? Journal of Reproductive Immunology. 2015;**109**:17-23

[19] Chernyshov VP, Tumanova LE, Sudoma IA, Bannikov VI. Th1 and Th2 in human IVF pregnancy with allogenic fetus. American Journal of Reproductive Immunology. 2008;**59**:352-358

[20] Tilburgs T, Roelen DL, Van der Mast BJ, De Groot-Swings GM, Kleijburg C, Scherjon SA, et al. Evidence for a selective migration of fetus-specific CD4+ CD25 bright regulatory T-cells from the peripheral blood to the deciduas in human pregnancy. Journal of Immunology. 2008;**180**(8):5737-5745

[21] Perni SC, Predanic M, Cho JE, Baergen RN. Placental pathology and pregnancy outcomes in donor and non-donor oocyte in vitro fertilization pregnancies. Journal of Perinatal Medicine. 2005;**33**:27-32

[22] Dietl J, Honig A, Kammerer U, Rieger L. Natural killer cells and dendritic cells at the human feto-maternal interface: An effective cooperation? Placenta. 2006;**27**:341-347

[23] Hiby SE, Walker JJ, O'shaughnessy KM, Redman CW, Carrington M, Trowsdale J, et al. Combinations of maternal KIR and fetal HLA-C genes influence the risk of preeclampsia and reproductive success. The Journal of Experimental Medicine. 2004;**200**:957-965

[24] Saito S, Shiozaki A, Sasaki Y, Nakashima A, Shima T, Ito M. Regulatory T cells and regulatory natural killer (NK) cells play important roles in feto-maternal tolerance. Seminars in Immunopathology. 2007;**29**:115-122

[25] Sauer MV. Defining the incidence of serious complications experienced by oocyte donors: A review of 1000 cases. American Journal of Obstetrics and Gynecology. 2001;**184**:277-278

[26] Girardi G, Yarilin D, Thurman JM, Holers VM, Salmon JE. Complement activation induces dysregulation of angiogenic factors and causes fetal rejection and growth restriction. The Journal of Experimental Medicine. 2006;**203**:2165-2175

[27] Albrecht ED, Pepe GJ. Estrogen regulation of placental angiogenesis and fetal ovarian development during primate pregnancy. The International Journal of Developmental Biology. 2010;**54**(2-3):397-408

[28] Pereira N, Elias RT, Christos PJ, Petrini AC, Hancock K, Lekovich JP, et al. Supraphysiologic estradiol is an

independent predictor of low birth weight in full-term singletons born after fresh embryo transfer. Human Reproduction. 2017;**32**(7):1410-1417. DOI: 10.1093/humrep/dex095

[29] Sindram-Trujillo AP, Scherjon SA, van Hulst-van Miert PP, van Schip JJ, Kanhai HH, Roelen DL, et al. Differential distribution of NK cells in decidua basalis compared with decidua parietalis after uncomplicated human term pregnancy. Human Immunology. 2003;**64**:921-929

[30] Le Bouteiller P, Pizzato N, Barakonyi A, Solier C. HLA-G, pre-eclampsia, immunity and vascular events. Journal of Reproductive Immunology. 2003;**59**:219-234

[31] Potnuru PP, Jefferies H, Lei R, Igwe P, Liang Y. Maternal pulmonary hypertension and cardiopulmonary outcomes during delivery hospitalization in the United States: A nationwide study from 2016-2020. Pregnancy Hypertension. 2024;**38**:101170. DOI: 10.1016/j.preghy.2024.101170. Epub 2024 Nov 18

Chapter 2

Endometrial Assessment to Ensure Successful Implantation

Tanya Timeva

Abstract

Most often, the term fertility preservation refers to options for storing genetic material such as eggs, spermatozoa, embryos or ovarian/testicular tissue. In order to achieve a subsequent pregnancy and childbirth, which is the main goal of methods in countries where surrogacy is not practiced, it is necessary to establish optimal conditions for preserving the uterus and its receptive tissue - in particular the endometrium. For this reason, the chapter discusses all methods for evaluating the endometrium in order to optimize the chances of pregnancy when using limited amounts of stored (frozen) genetic material. It is of utmost importance for patients to ensure the best conditions for embryo transfer, with the highest rate of achieving implantation and pregnancy. The methods used in practice for endometrial evaluation can be summarized and grouped into:

- Evaluation of the anatomical features of the endometrial thickness and the uterine cavity (ultrasound, Doppler, hysteroscopy, MRI);
- Evaluation of function of the endometrium (endometrial biopsy, receptivity test, microbiome);
- Additional methods like hormonal and immunological and in case of deviations, to suggest procedures that increase success rates.

Keywords: endometrium, implantation, EMT, IVF/ICSI-ET, ultrasound

1. Introduction

The various fertility preservation methods raise numerous questions that must be addressed when attempting to achieve pregnancy at a later stage. Depending on the specific reasons for fertility preservation—social, medical, or other—and especially on the age of the patients, this chapter will discuss how to optimize conditions for achieving pregnancy using assisted reproductive technologies in a female population. A key step for a successful pregnancy is creating favorable conditions for the implantation process. The main "players" in this process are the embryo, developed to the stage of hatching blastocyst, and the receptive endometrium.

Despite the cutting-edge innovations in the pharmaceutical industry, advancements in embryology lab techniques, developments in genetics and immunology, and the optimization of cryopreservation methods in recent years, reported success rates from

European registries (e.g., for the year 2019) indicate: when freeze-all cycles were not considered for the calculations, the clinical PRs per aspiration were 28.5 and 26.2% for IVF and ICSI, respectively. After FET with embryos originating from own eggs, the PR per thawing was at 35.1% and with embryos originating from donated eggs at 43.0% [1].

Trying to achieve optimal success rates after ART, the task of reproductive specialists for patients who have undergone gamete/embryo/reproductive tissue cryopreservation is to create conditions for a live birth, especially for those patients who, after treatment, are unable to restore their reproductive capacity, particularly their gamete production. Efforts are primarily directed at monitoring and preparing the endometrium for subsequent implantation, based on the physiological characteristics of its cyclical development.

2. Basic concepts and dynamic changes in the endometrium

The endometrium is the inner epithelial lining of the uterine cavity, structurally composed of a basal and a functional layer. Its thickness varies depending on the phases of the menstrual cycle and undergoes cyclic regeneration. At the end of the desquamation phase, the endometrium consists only of its basal layer, measuring approximately 1–2 mm (lamina baslis **B, Figure 1**). Estrogens, whose secretion intensifies after day 3 of the menstrual cycle, stimulate the proliferation of all structural components of the endometrium—loose connective tissue, blood vessels, tubular glands, and surface epithelium. By the end of the proliferative phase, the endometrial thickness reaches approximately 7–8 mm. The onset of ovulation, the formation of the corpus luteum, and its progesterone production induce changes in the epithelial cells, stromal cells, matrix, and blood vessels and contribute to the morphological formation of the remaining layers: compact outer layer (stratum compactum) and intermediate layer (stratum spongiosum) (C, S, **Figure 1**).

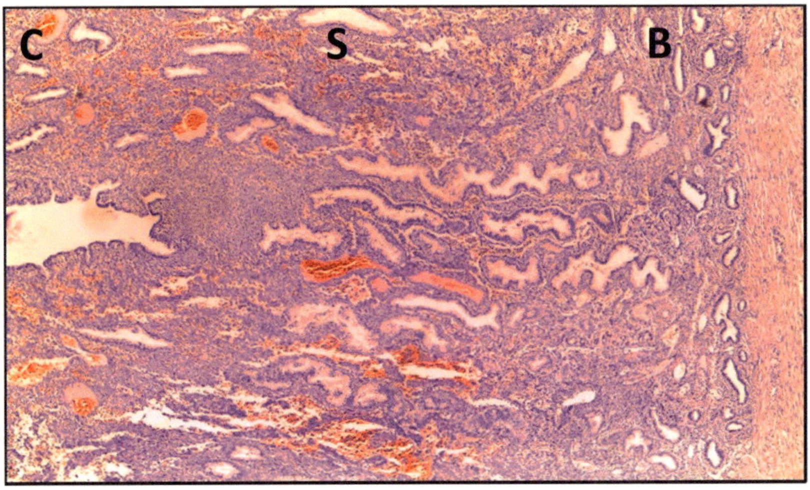

C - compact layer; **S** - spongy layer; **B** - lamina basalis

Figure 1.
Endometrium in the mid-secretory phase (histological preparation by Drenski R.) C - compact layer; S - spongy layer; B - lamina basalis.

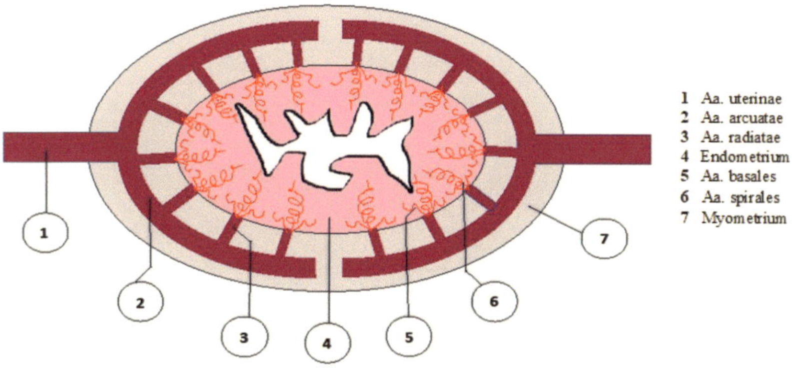

Figure 2.
Schematic of endometrial vascularization (diagram by Golemanova N.)

We use the term decidualization to describe this remodeling process, which, in addition to phenotypic cellular changes and angiogenesis, is characterized by the dominance of so-called uterine NK cells. The formation of the decidua in humans is still not fully understood. It is hypothesized that decidualization can occur not only during pregnancy but also as a result of prolonged progesterone exposure or can be influenced by the expression profile of different receptors as progesterone receptor membrane component 1 (PGRMC1) [2–4]. During this process, stromal cells transform into cells that secrete specific factors such as prolactin, insulin-like growth factor binding protein-1 (IGFBP-1), and vascular endothelial growth factor (VEGF), among others [5, 6]. Prostaglandins secreted by decidual cells also play a role in the complex interactions among progesterone, prolactin, relaxin, cytokines, and growth factors. Some authors even describe the endometrium as a "dynamic endocrine organ" with a central role in the implantation process [7].

Blood supply to the endometrium is of critical importance for the implantation process and subsequent placentation. The diagram below (**Figure 2**) schematically illustrates the uterine arteries (aa. uterinae) and their arcuate branches (aa. arcuatae), followed by radial arteries (aa. radiatae), and their terminal branches (spiral and basal arteries—aa. spirales and aa. basales), reaching the various layers of the endometrium. Hormonal factors influence the innervation of the uterine arteries, both cholinergic and adrenergic, and regulate the spontaneous contractile activity of the smooth muscle in the vessel walls. The smaller branches of the uterine arteries are most densely innervated, which is why vasoconstrictors such as vasopressin, endothelin, oxytocin, and norepinephrine have the strongest effect on these vessels [8]. This supports the logical application of vasodilators (e.g., nitrocompounds, phosphodiesterase-5 inhibitors) to enhance blood flow and improve conditions for implantation.

3. Methods for assessing the endometrium

3.1 Classification of methods

In clinical practice, a variety of methods are used to assess the structure and function of the uterine lining (**Table 1**).

The earliest methods for assessing the endometrium date back to 1950, when the first issue of Fertility and Sterility published Noyes' landmark study on endometrial dating *via*

Type	Methods
Imaging (non-invasive)	Ultrasound, 3D, Doppler, MRI
Invasive	Histological
	Hysteroscopic – diagnostic and/or operative for: polyps, septum, fibroids, adhesions, tubal occlusion (hydrosalpinx), etc.
Laboratory	Immunological
	Genetic

Table 1.
Summary of methods for endometrial assessment.

biopsy [9]. This is perhaps one of the most frequently cited methodological articles when discussing the role of the endometrium in infertility. It examined histological changes in the endometrium through photomicrographs and clinical correlation with the menstrual cycle day in 300 women. There are various methods for obtaining endometrial biopsies for histological examination. For the sole purpose of "dating," aspiration techniques using an atraumatic catheter are preferred. The procedure is done on an outpatient basis and without anesthesia. However, due to the availability of advanced ultrasound diagnostics and detailed hormonal profiling, this method is now used less frequently.

Furthermore, it is increasingly recognized that a morphologically normal endometrium does not invariably indicate a receptive state. Therefore, it is advisable to employ the full range of currently available diagnostic modalities for endometrial assessment, particularly in patients with recurrent implantation failure (RIF).

3.2 Ultrasound evaluation of the endometrium

Ultrasound monitoring of endometrial development is a noninvasive, easily performed, and widely applied method for all patients desiring pregnancy. It is of fundamental importance in donor programs for the proper timing of both fresh and frozen embryo transfers (ET). The dynamic cellular processes in the endometrial glands, stroma, and blood vessels present typical sonographic characteristics and images. Additionally, some authors suggest the possibility of cycle-to-cycle variation [10].

Ultrasound evaluation of the endometrium includes measuring its thickness, determining its echogenicity (pattern), characterizing vascularization (with Doppler), and identifying pathological abnormalities in the uterine cavity, such as polyps, submucosal fibroids, and so on. Modern ultrasound equipment and the capabilities of 3D sonography allow the calculation of uterine cavity volume.

Some authors divide endometrial evaluation indicators into anatomical (thickness and pattern) and functional (TV-color Doppler: S/D, PI, RI) parameters [11]. The use of multiple combined parameters has led to the development of composite evaluation systems, such as the uterine ultrasonographic scoring system [12], similar to scoring systems used in other OB/GYN subspecialties.

3.2.1 Endometrial thickness

Meta-analyses on this topic identify endometrial thickness (EMT) as a leading sonographic indicator [13, 14]. Precision measurement involves a transvaginal ultrasound transducer with a 5 MHz frequency and a frozen gray-scale image on the longitudinal axis of the uterus. EMT is defined as the maximum anterior-posterior distance between the echogenic boundaries of the endometrial-myometrial junction [10]. There is ongoing debate in the literature about the significance of a thin endometrium and its association with lower implantation rates during IVF procedures. This raises questions about threshold values—the minimal and maximal EMT at which ET should be reconsidered or avoided. Results across studies show conflicting data regarding the correlation between pregnancy outcomes and EMT [15–20]. The validity of conclusions depends on study design, patient population (age, inclusion/exclusion criteria), stimulation protocols, sample size, and statistical methods. A comprehensive meta-analysis by Kasius et al. [13] published in Human Reproduction Update included 10,724 women across 22 cohort studies. An sROC analysis revealed no clear discriminatory capacity of EMT for predicting pregnancy. A thin endometrium (≤7 mm) was present in only 2.4% of reported cases (260/10724). In this group, lower clinical pregnancy and live birth rates were observed [OR 0.38 (95% CI 0.09–1.5)]. Clinical pregnancy rates were 23.3% for EMT ≤7 mm vs. 48.1% for EMT >7 mm [OR 0.42 (95% CI 0.27–0.67)] with positive predictive value 77% and negative predictive value 48%. These findings indicate that EMT has limited capacity to identify women with low pregnancy potential after IVF. The commonly reported lower threshold of 7 mm is associated with decreased success but is relatively rare. Another recent retrospective analysis has been conducted on two randomized phase III clinical trials carried out in Europe and America, involving a total of n = 1401 patients aged 18–42, BMI <30 kg/m^2, <3 previous ART attempts, and ≥ 3 aspirated oocytes after COH with GnRH-agonist or GnRH-antagonist protocol [21]. The endometrial lining was measured on the day of ET, and patients were divided into groups as follows: EMT ≤ 8 mm, n = 117 (8.35%), EMT 8–15 mm, n = 1200 (85.65%), and EMT > 15 mm, n = 84 (6%). The predictive value of EMT was tested for each millimeter, and it was found that at a threshold ≥9 mm, the probability of pregnancy was higher compared to patients with EMT of 3–8 mm (odds ratio (OR) = 1.69, 95% CI: 1.23–2.35, p = 0.001; sensitivity 88.89%, specificity 17.52%, positive predictive value 39.02%, negative predictive value 72.64%). In multivariate regression analysis, after controlling for attempt, women's age, and the number of oocytes, EMT was a statistically significant predictor of live birth (OR = 1.05, 95% CI: 1.00–1.10, P = 0.0351). If EMT is indeed an independent factor influencing outcomes, these data suggest that with a baseline birth rate of 20%, an increase of 2 mm in EMT should lead to an increase in birth rate by ~1.6%. The final conclusion of the authors is that EMT can be ignored in most patients; only extreme values deserve further diagnostic workup. It must be made very clear that in most publications concerning EMT and clinical pregnancies and live births, patients with intrauterine pathology such as endometrial polyps, submucosal or intramural myomas, intrauterine adhesions, septum, and so forth are excluded. Some of the mentioned are demonstrated below on **Figures 3** and **4**.

Further in-depth research is needed on the independent predictive value of the endometrial lining. Success rates are influenced by many factors that have a complex impact, such as the woman's age, number of aspirated oocytes, E2 levels, and embryo quality. The analysis of results for EMT when comparing pregnant and nonpregnant groups shows a significantly larger diameter of the uterine lining in pregnant women (10.6 ± 1.8 vs. 9.9 ± 1.8 mm) (p < 0.01) [22]. Interesting data are reported in another large study by Holden et al. from 2017 [23]. Included in the study were 6331 patients with their first attempt and fresh ET, with EMT determined on the day of ovulation timing. The thinnest endometrium observed with pregnancy was 3.7 mm, and the thickest endometrium was 27 mm, both resulting in live births. The author collective did not find an association between EMT and the level of spontaneous abortions (RR: 0.99; 95% CI: 0.91–1.07), unlike other teams where reported data indicate a dependence

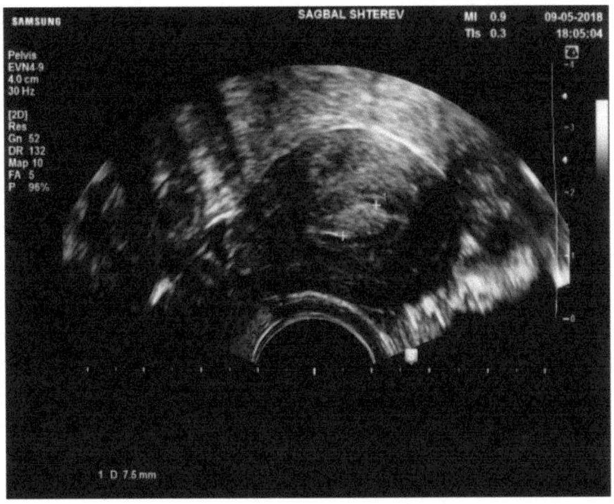

Figure 3.
Endometrial polyp.

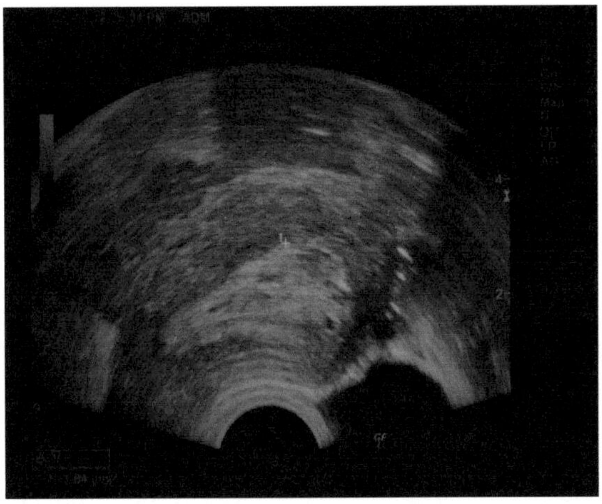

Figure 4.
Hyperplastic endometrium.

of spontaneous abortion and ectopic pregnancy rates on EMT [24, 25]. Wu et al. make conclusions based on 2106 ETs and find that spontaneous abortions are more frequent in women with EMT below 7 mm, while Yuan's team finds an ectopic pregnancy rate of 24.5% in women with EMT < 8 mm compared to 13.6% in those with EMT ≥ 8 mm. As a discussion point, it can be noted that with insufficiently prepared or functioning endometrium, the risk of obstetric complications increases, so it is important whether a spontaneous cycle or hormone replacement therapy will be preferred in patients planning pregnancy/ET after cryopreservation for fertility preservation purposes.

3.2.2 Endometrial pattern (type and echogenicity)

In addition to thickness, the endometrial pattern (echogenicity) is an important characteristic. A triple-line (trilaminar) appearance indicates good estrogenization. After this pattern is observed (typically at ovulatory E2 peak), the endometrium transitions into the

Pattern	Ultrasound characteristics
A	Triple-line central hyperechoic line surrounded by two hypoechoic layers
B	An intermediate isoechogenic with the same reflectivity as the surrounding myometrium and a poorly defined central echogenic line
C	Homogenous, hyperechogenic endometrium

Table 2.
Different types of endometrium based on echogenicity [27].

secretory phase, becoming progressively more echogenic. However, comparisons across studies are complicated by the use of different classification systems. In an earlier study, Sher et al. divided endometrial types into two echogenic patterns: grade I and grade II [26]. Zhao and colleagues studied 3319 women and divided the patients according to the type of endometrium as presented in **Table 2**. However, the relationship between echogenicity and successful implantation is complex and not always straightforward.

From the conclusions of the authors, it becomes clear that conditions such as recurrent early and late abortions, preterm births, and delayed intrauterine fetal growth may partly be associated with poor endometrial preparation for implantation. Of course, isolated influence of the endometrium on the development of pregnancy is difficult to prove, as there is a complex set of factors directly related to successful outcomes. According to Coelho et al., the percentage of clinical pregnancies with a thin endometrium under 7 mm is high in women who have retrieved over 7 oocytes or have over 4 developing embryos [28]. This means that ovarian response is a better prognostic factor than a thin endometrium, especially in young women freezing eggs for delaying motherhood. According to the same author collective, in women with diminished ovarian reserve, a thin endometrium is encountered more frequently compared to endometrium with normal thickness (17/57 (30%) vs. 80/460 (17%), respectively, P = 0.03). Widely adopted in Bulgaria and used in daily clinical practice is classification of type of uterine lining, proposed by Shterev At [29]. Postmenstrually, in the early follicular phase, the uterine lining appears as a *line*, which we call type "*L*". In the late follicular phase, the endometrium has a trilinear structure and resembles a *mussel shell*; hence, it is defined as type "*M*". In the early and intermediate luteal phase, the uterine lining becomes denser, hyperechoic, and resembles a bag filled with pebbles or *sand* – "*S*". This lining is classified as type "S1"—with thickening only on the lateral lines, and "S2"—completely hyperechoic, characteristic of the late luteal phase. Any ultrasound examination outside the specified parameters should be marked with "X," and additional methods of investigation should be used, as ultrasonography is insufficient regarding oncodiagnostics. All pathological deviations are visualized most clearly in the late follicular phase of the cycle, when maximum endometrial thickness is achieved. Here, it is worth noting an interesting fact about the ultrasound examination of uterine lining type *"M" (mussel shell)*, demonstrated in the presented images (**Figures 5** and **6**).

The different echogenicity of tissues is explained by the greater fluid content within them, suggesting that in the presented cases, the morphological substrate of the functional layer of the endometrium is differently prepared or hormonally influenced. Whether certain ultrasound characteristics of the uterine lining are associated with greater receptivity will be the subject of future studies. Today, in clinical practice, upon encountering specific ultrasound findings, diagnostic clarification is preferred before proceeding with ET. Such cases include diagnosing, for example, endometrial polyps, hyperplastic growths, or other pathologies (**Figures 3** and **4**).

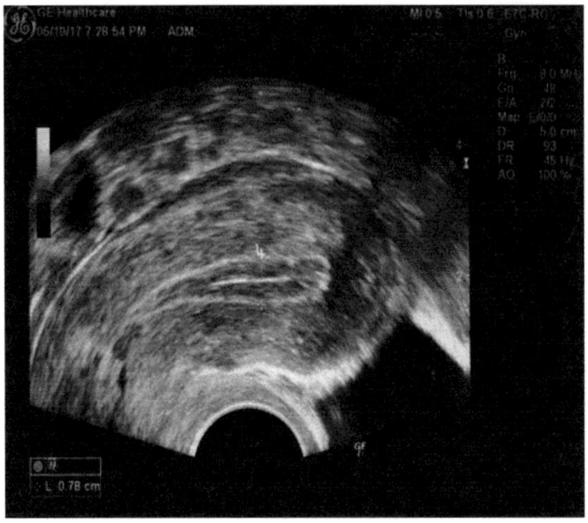

Figure 5.
Endometrium type "M" with similar echogenicity to the myometrium.

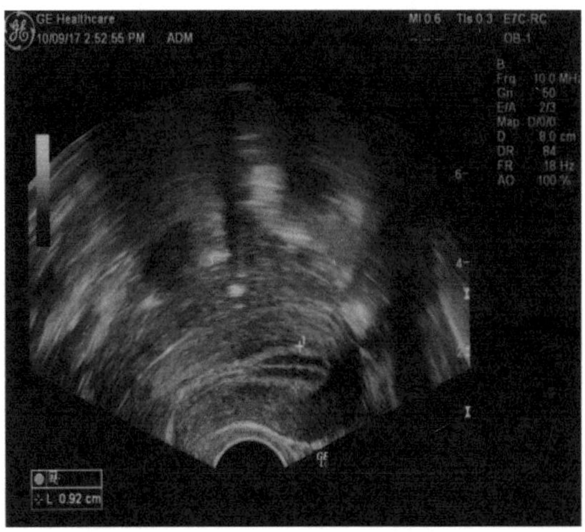

Figure 6.
Endometrium type "M" hypoechoic compared to the myometrium.

3.2.3 Blood supply

Another important indicator in assessing the endometrium during ultrasound examination is the adequacy of its vascularization, evaluated through various types of Doppler: color, pulsed, and continuous (**Figures** 7 and **8**). Zhang et al. conduct 3D ultrasound measurement on the day of hCG, combined with color Doppler examination (S/D, RI, PI) and 3D PDUS histogram analysis to calculate endometrial volume and vascularization indices (VI, FI, VFI) [30]. The publication considers seven indicators: EMT, type (echogenicity) of the endometrium, uterine contractions for 2 minutes, Doppler of the uterine artery, power Doppler of the endometrium (do the vascular zones reach the basal layer), myometrial power Doppler, and echogenicity. The 562 examined women are divided into groups based on the mentioned indicators, but no significant difference in pregnancy rates was observed. Despite the

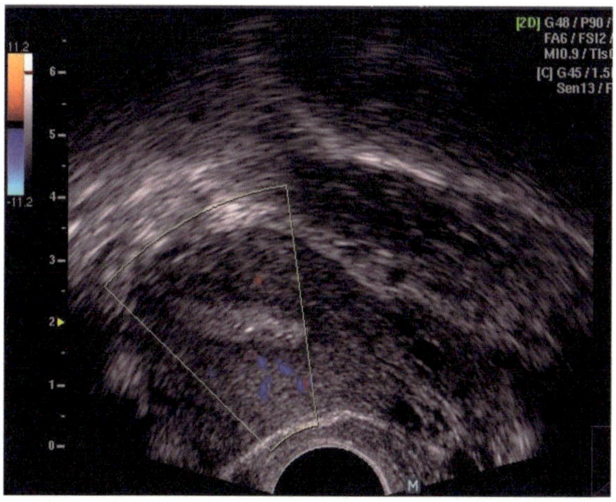

Figure 7.
Demonstration of vascularization using color Doppler of subendometrial zone.

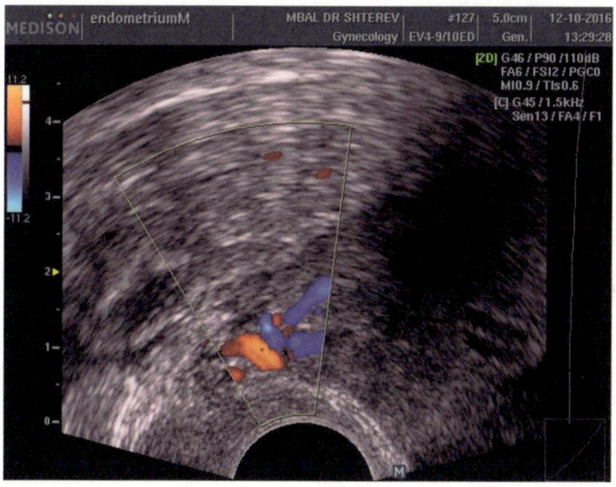

Figure 8.
Transvaginal color Doppler of a. uterina.

comprehensive assessment, the authors conclude that it cannot identify the population of patients with altered endometrial receptivity.

To the planned markers for examination, the indices of ovarian stromal vessels can also be added, and an investigation of VEGF can be conducted. With the accumulation of sufficient results, the Doppler characteristics of spiral arteries could be interpreted in relation to the development of complications during pregnancy, such as preeclampsia, fetal growth retardation, elevated blood pressure, and others. This would be beneficial for predicting the development and outcome of pregnancy and represents a step forward in preconception care for patients.

Using all the possibilities of ultrasound equipment, an evaluation can also be made of the peristaltic waves of the myometrium, which depend on the day of the cycle and the duration of progesterone substitution. On the **Table 3** below, some ultrasound characteristics of the endometrium that favor implantation are presented, thus making an optimal choice for the day of ET.

Studied parameter	Values on transvaginal ultrasound
Endometrial thickness	>7 mm
Color Doppler indices of subendometrial	Pulsatality Index <1.25
Blood flow in Zone III	Refractory Index <0.6
Assessment of myometrial peristaltic waves	When more than 4 waves/min - need for prolonged progesterone exposure

Table 3.
Ultrasound characteristics of the endometrium favoring implantation [31].

The application of additional ultrasound techniques, including Doppler examination, does not require special qualifications and is performed quickly. Despite the low prognostic value in certain patients, it could aid in an adequate therapeutic approach and optimal conditions for achieving pregnancy. **Figures 9** and **10** demonstrate various Doppler assessments for selecting the appropriate time for ET.

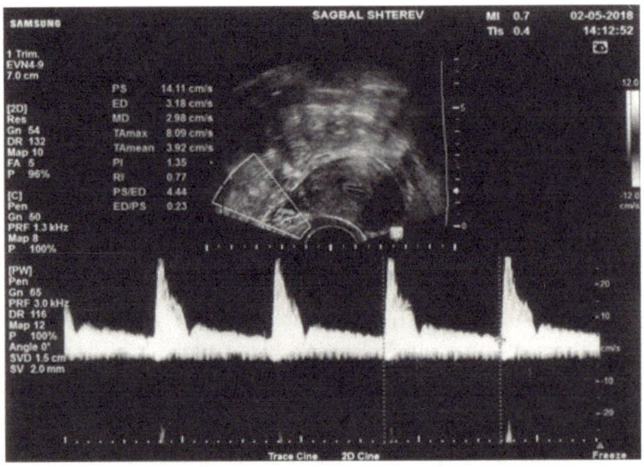

Figure 9.
Pulsed Doppler.

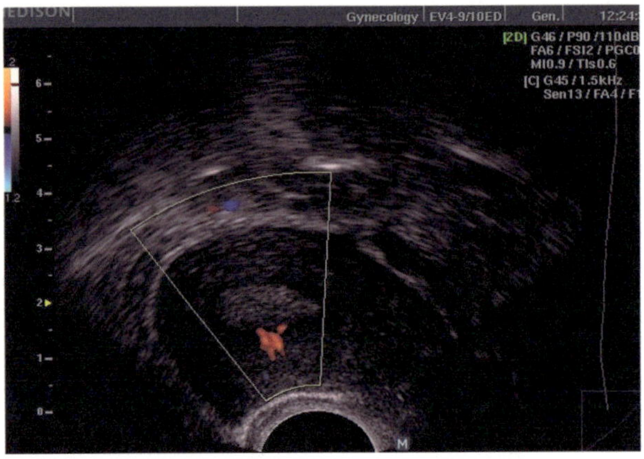

Figure 10.
Color Doppler.

3.2.4 Limitations of ultrasound assessment

While ultrasound is a useful tool, it has its limitations. It cannot assess the molecular and genetic readiness of the endometrium. Receptivity is determined at a cellular level by the expression of hundreds of genes, which is impossible to visualize with ultrasound. For this reason, more invasive methods exist, such as endometrial biopsy and molecular tests (e.g., ERA test), which provide more precise information about the "implantation window."

3.3 The role of hysteroscopy as a diagnostic and therapeutic procedure

Through the hysteroscopic method, direct visualization and assessment of the endometrium, its blood supply, and various pathological processes, including the size and shape of the uterine cavity, are achieved. Some authors describe a wide range of 18–50% of recorded uterine pathology in patients before IVF, with or without recurrent implantation failures, and without prior suspicion of anomalies [32, 33]. A higher incidence of adhesions has been described in patients with a history of curettage or uterine surgery [34]. Let us emphasize, however, that in cases of fertility preservation, a high incidence of uterine pathology should not be expected, as this is not a population with infertility of various etiologies.

The hysteroscopic method serves simultaneously for assessment, diagnostic examination with biopsy, and treatment, including surgical intervention. Cutting with scissors is preferred over electrosurgery to avoid thermal effects and endometrial damage [35]. Various theories are discussed regarding the favorable influence of hysteroscopy on the success rate in a subsequent attempt. On one hand, a smooth ET is guaranteed due to passage through the cervical canal, and on the other hand, a favorable impact on endometrial receptivity is assumed through mechanical hysteroscopic manipulation and distension of the cavity.

3.4 Immunological methods

According to Sarani et al. [36], the most pronounced morphological changes in the endometrium are observed around day 6 after the onset of the LH-peak. Buscher et al. [37] earlier determined, by examining serum HCG concentration, that implantation in pregnancies resulting in live birth occurred between day 5.9 and 7.5 after follicular puncture [36, 37]. From this, we should conclude that optimal planning of the embryo transfer (ET) day is crucial for patients who have cryopreserved embryos or oocytes. The maximum receptivity of the uterine lining is characterized by the expression of various endometrial products, some of which are well-studied. These include integrins, Interleukin-1 (IL-1), Leukemia Inhibitory Factor (LIF), Colony Stimulating Factor-1 (CSF-1), Transmembrane Mucin (MUC-1), Trophinin, L-selectin, and Wnt family members [38, 39]. These substances control the processes of adhesion to the endometrial epithelium and also participate in the division and differentiation of embryonic cells. Such substances can therefore be used as biomarkers for endometrial receptivity [40]. Molecular deviations at the endometrial level and disturbances in the embryo-endometrial dialog are at the root of cases with recurrent IVF/ICSI failures [41]. The role of CA-125 as a potential marker for endometrial receptivity in assisted reproduction has also been studied, but no correlation with treatment outcome has been found [42].

Before the widespread adoption of genetic testing, Acosta et al. [43] dated the implantation window by examining serum concentrations of LH, E2, and P, along with vaginal ultrasound and endometrial biopsies [43]. More recently, methods have been introduced into practice that analyze endometrial fluid, and conclusions about its receptivity are drawn from its specific profile [44–48]. Leading specialists in this field of innovative endometrial research and its functional characteristics are from Fundacio'n Instituto Valenciano de Infertilidad, Valencia, Spain, under the guidance of Prof. Carlos Simon and Prof. Antonio Pellicer. The advantage of analyzing endometrial fluid is that the method is practically noninvasive. For instance, these authors have demonstrated that prostaglandins (PGE2 and PGF2α) determine the implantation window. The target patient group for such investigations is precisely women with RIF. Other teams have found that various components of the prostaglandin system, such as cyclooxygenase-2 (COX-2), secretory phospholipase A2 group: IIA, V, and IB (sPLA2-IIA, sPLA2-V, and sPLA2-IB), glypican-1, PG-E synthase, PG-E receptors, and lysophosphatidic acid receptor 3 (LPA3), are present in significantly lower concentrations in 85% of couples with RIF [49].

For both preimplantation and recurrent postimplantation losses, thorough investigations of T-helper (Th) cells and specifically their subgroups (Th1, Th2, Th17, and T-regulatory (Treg) cells), as well as Natural Killer (NK) cells, are necessary [50]. Published evidence of immune changes in these cases will identify patient subgroups most likely to benefit from immunomodulatory therapies for a successful pregnancy. The regulation of the immune response during pregnancy has been studied for a long time, and data demonstrate the involvement of steroid hormones P and E through their influence on apoptosis and the cytokine profile of mDCs (monocyte-derived dendritic cells) [51].

Additional information regarding the intricate mechanisms of the implantation process can also be obtained from *in vitro* studies on human endometrial cells or cultures of human trophoblasts and placental tissues. N. Macklon used a human co-culture model, consisting of decidualized endometrial stromal cells and single hatching blastocysts, to identify the soluble factors involved in the implantation process and subsequent embryonic development [52]. This practically means an attempt to "imitate" the phases of the implantation process and identify the mediators involved in the dialog between the embryo and the endometrium. Researchers have found that incorrect decidualization can lead to the implantation of a "suboptimal embryo", and the expected result may be a spontaneous pregnancy loss. This sheds new light on the determining role of the endometrium as one of the possible causes of recurrent miscarriages. Research on Apo A-I is also of interest. It has been identified as an anti-implantation protein secreted by the differentiating endometrium, and higher expression is found in ectopic secretory endometrium in patients with endometriosis. Thus, a disruption in Apo A-1 secretion could be an important factor in the pathogenesis of endometriosis and crucial for clarifying the mechanisms of RIF [53].

There is growing evidence that endometrial function in the stimulated cycle is adversely affected by supraphysiological estrogen levels and premature progesterone secretion, leading to immunological dysregulation of the endometrium and subsequent implantation failure [54–56]. Furthermore, "omics" technologies have been used as a molecular tool to determine the effects of stimulating protocols on endometrial gene expression and clinical outcome [57].

3.5 Genetic methods

The expression of numerous human endometrial genes has been investigated during different phases of the menstrual cycle in fertile and infertile women using transcriptomic methods. Endometrial biopsies were performed, and based on the results processed through bioinformatics, an Endometrial Receptivity Array (ERA) test was developed, which can be applied in clinical practice [58]. The test evaluates 238 selected genes, and their up- or downregulation determines the optimal period for implantation with high specificity (Sp = 0.8857) and sensitivity (Se = 0.99758). The ERA test is a reliable method for determining the precise timing of the Window of Implantation (WOI) and holds an advantage over histological dating of endometrial receptivity [59]. When endometrial receptivity in RIF patients is identified using the ERA test, and embryo transfers are performed according to the ERA data, a 62.8% pregnancy rate is achieved. The authors have developed a clinical algorithm that enables the application of personalized embryo transfer for RIF patients [60].

Recently, data from a study on the Human Gene Expression Endometrial Receptivity database (HGEx-ERdb), which contains 19,285 genes, have been reported. It was shown that 179 genes can be identified as Receptivity-Associated Genes (RAGs), which are useful for determining endometrial receptivity [61]. This approach offers new perspectives for researchers, but there is still a long way to go before its implementation in clinical practice.

For these research methods, the most relevant group comprises patients with recurrent failures, because it is precisely in these patients that gene array methods discover altered gene expression. More than 90% of the genes were downregulated, and these are involved in regulating three main pathways: the cell cycle, cell-to-cell contact, and the Wnt pathway. On the other hand, at least two genes, “Slug” and “DKK1,” were upregulated. The DKK1 gene is known as a potent inhibitor of the Wnt pathway and is a proapoptotic agent. It is evident that there’s a general dysregulation of gene expression in the endometrium of RIF patients, but the clinical significance of all changes in gene expression has not yet been proven [62].

The same research group continues to investigate changes in microRNA profiles in the endometrium of RIF patients. MicroRNAs are known as posttranscriptional regulators of gene expression involved in a range of physiological and pathological events. Recently, it has been reported that at least 13 miRNAs are expressed quite specifically in endometrial samples, with 10 of them being upregulated and 3 miRNAs downregulated. Since specifically expressed miRNAs appear to regulate over 3800 genes, subsequent experiments assessing miRNA levels show that members of cell-adhesive molecules, the Wnt signaling pathway, and cell cycles are lower in RIF patients [49].

It is clear that microarray techniques are highly sensitive and informative, but the obtained data are difficult to interpret as clinically significant parameters and criteria. New developments in oncotherapy, as well as the impact of applied therapeutic regimens on the molecular mechanisms of various ongoing processes in the body, including implantation, should also be considered.

4. Discussion

More information and recommendations on female fertility preservation for women with cancer, benign diseases, and also transgender patients and women undergoing elective freezing will be covered in the ESHRE guideline on female fertility preservation (www.eshre.eu/FFPguideline) [63]. When preserving fertility for social reasons, no significant changes in the endometrium are expected, apart from age-related alterations. In modern reproductive medicine, the “freeze-all” strategy has entered clinical practice and established itself as a highly successful approach for achieving pregnancy in general IVF population. Therefore, it can definitively be asserted that the achievements and practices leading to pregnancy, considering endometrial preparation whether natural cycles (NCs) lead to a higher live birth rate after the first FET cycle compared to hormone replacement therapy (HRT) cycles in women with a regular ovulatory cycle, can also be translated to the population undergoing fertility preservation treatment [64]. Cases involving hormone-dependent tumors can be considered more unique. In such instances, treatment is conducted by a multidisciplinary team. Onco-therapy can have various effects on the endometrium depending on the type of treatment, dose, duration, and the patient's individual reaction. Here are the main ways in which different types of onco-therapy can affect the endometrium:

- If radiation therapy targets the pelvic area, then we can observe thinning and drying of the lining due to damage to blood vessels and glands and formation of connective tissue, which can lead to narrowing of the uterine cavity or adhesions and reduced elasticity.

- Some chemotherapy drugs can affect ovarian function, leading to reduced estrogen and progesterone production. This can result in amenorrhea due to endometrial atrophy or irregular cycle. Although the endometrium is not a primary target of chemotherapy, some drugs can affect rapidly dividing cells, including those in the endometrium, which can lead to inflammation or changes in the lining.

- Hormone therapy is frequently used for hormone-sensitive tumors (e.g., Tamoxifen) While Tamoxifen acts as an anti-estrogen in the breast, it can act as an estrogen in the endometrium. This can lead to endometrial hyperplasia or unusual vaginal bleeding. GnRH agonists suppress hormone production by the ovaries, leading to temporary menopause and endometrial atrophy.

It is crucial to always discuss potential side effects with the treating physician, as individual reactions can vary, and strategies exist to manage or reduce these adverse reactions.

5. Conclusion

Translating all scientifically validated approaches—originally developed for treating infertile patients—to the population of women planning pregnancy after fertility preservation can help achieve optimal rates of clinical pregnancies and live births. However, over-medicalization should be avoided. Most patients undergoing fertility preservation are not infertile, and in many cases, we are dealing with healthy individuals seeking to delay childbearing due to personal or medical reasons. The ideal study model for evaluating endometrial function remains the recurrent implantation failure (RIF) population, although recent debates have raised concerns that this condition may be overdiagnosed.

Author details

Tanya Timeva[1,2]*

1 IVF Department, SAGBAL "D-r Shterev", Sofia, Bulgaria

2 Ruse University "Angel Kunchev", Ruse, Bulgaria

*Address all correspondence to: ttimeva@yahoo.com

References

[1] The European IVF Monitoring Consortium (EIM) for the European Society of Human Reproduction and Embryology (ESHRE), Smeenk J, Wyns C, De Geyter C, et al. ART in Europe, 2019: Results generated from European registries by ESHRE. Human Reproduction. 2023;**38**(12):2321-2338. DOI: 10.1093/humrep/dead197

[2] Dunn C, Kelly R, Critchley H. Decidualization of the human endometrial stromal cell: An enigmatic transformation. Reproductive Biomedicine Online. 2003;**7**:151-161

[3] Kennedy T, Gillio-Meina C, Phang SH. Prostaglandins and the initiation of blastocyst implantation and decidualization. Reproduction. 2007;**134**:635-643

[4] Liu H, Franken A, Bielfeld AP, et al. Progesterone-induced progesterone receptor membrane component 1 rise-to-decline changes are essential for decidualization. Reproductive Biology and Endocrinology. 2024;**22**:20. DOI: 10.1186/s12958-024-01188-9

[5] Richards RG, Rar AK, Frank GR, Hartman SM, Jikihara H. Fibroblast cells from term human decidua closely resemble endometrial stromal cells: Induction of prolactin and insulin-like growth factor binding protein-1 expression. Biology of Reproduction. 1995;**52**:609-615

[6] Sugino N, Kashida S, Karube-Harada A, Takiguchi S, Kato H. Expression of vascular endothelial growth factor VEGF and its receptors in human endometrium throughout the menstrual cycle and in early pregnancy. Reproduction. 2002;**123**:379-387

[7] Banker M, Gupte-Shah A. Effect of ovarian stimulation on the endometrium. In: Principles and Practice of Controlled Ovarian Stimulation in ART. New Delhi: Springer; 2015. DOI: 10.1007/978-81-322-1686-5_21

[8] Akerlund M. Vascularization of human endometrium. Uterine blood flow in healthy condition and in primary dysmenorrhoea. Annals of the New York Academy of Sciences. 1994;**30**(734):47-56

[9] Noyes RW, Hertig AT, Rock J. Dating the endometrial biopsy. Fertility and Sterility. 1950;**1**:3-25

[10] Basir GS, O WS, WWK S, EHY N, Ho PC. Evaluation of cycle-to-cycle variation of endometrial responsiveness using transvaginal sonography in women undergoing assisted reproduction. Ultrasound in Obstetrics & Gynecology. 2002;**19**:484-489

[11] Friedler S, Schenker J, Herman A, Lewin A. The role of ultrasonography in the evaluation of endometrial receptivity following assisted reproductive treatments: A critical review. Human Reproduction Update. 1996;**2**(4):323-335

[12] Baruffi R, Contart P, Mauri A, Petersen C, Felipe V, Garbellini E, et al. Uterine Ultrasonographic scoring system as a method for the prognosis of embryo implantation. Journal of Assisted Reproduction and Genetics. 2002;**19**:99-102

[13] Kasius A, Smit J, Torrance H, Marinus JC, Mol EBW, Opmeer BC, et al. Endometrial thickness and pregnancy rates after IVF: A systematic review and meta-analysis. Human Reproduction Update. 2014;**20**(4):530-541

[14] Momeni M, Rahbar M, Kovanci E. A meta-analysis of the relationship between endometrial thickness and outcome of in vitro fertilization cycle. Journal of Human Reproductive Sciences. 2011;**4**(3):130-137

[15] Noyes N, Liu HC, Sultan K, Schattman G, Rosenwaks Z. Endometrial thickness appears to be a significant factor in embryo implantation in in-vitro fertilization. Human Reproduction. 1995;**10**:919-922

[16] Rinaldi L, Lisi F, Floccari A, Lisi R, Pepe G, Fishel S. Endometrial thickness as a predictor of pregnancy after in-vitro fertilization but not after intracytoplasmic sperm injection. Human Reproduction. 1996;**11**:1538-1541

[17] Yuval Y, Lipitz S, Dor J, Achiron R. The relationships between endometrial thickness, and blood flow and pregnancy rates in in-vitro fertilization. Human Reproduction. 1999;**14**:1067-1071

[18] De Geyter C, Schmitter M, De Geyter M, Nieschlag E, Holzgreve W, Schneider HP. Prospective evaluation of the ultrasound appearance of the endometrium in a cohort of 1,186 infertile women. Fertility and Sterility. 2000;**73**:106-113

[19] Bassil S. Changes in endometrial thickness, thickness, length and pattern in predicting pregnancy outcome during ovarian stimulation in in vitro fertilization. Ultrasound in Obstetrics & Gynecology. 2001;**18**:258-263

[20] Kovacs P, Matyas S, Boda K, Kaali SG. The effect of endometrial thickness on IVF/ICSI outcome. Human Reproduction. 2003;**18**:2337-2341

[21] Griesinger G, Trevisan S, Cometti B. Endometrial thickness on the day of embryo transfer is a poor predictor of IVF treatment outcome. Human Reproduction Open. 29 Jan 2018;**2018**(1):hox031. DOI: 10.1093/hropen/hox031

[22] Fang R, Cai L, Xiong F, Chen J, Yang W, Zhao X. The effect of endometrial thickness on the day of hCG administration on pregnancy outcome in the first fresh IVF/ICSI cycle. Gynecological Endocrinology. 2016;**32**(6):473-476

[23] Holden E, Laura E, Dodge R, Sneeringer V, Moragianni A, Penzias S, et al. Thicker endometrial linings are associated with better IVF outcomes: A cohort of 6331 women. Human Fertility. 2018;**21**(4):288-293. DOI: 10.1080/14647273.2017.1334130

[24] Yuan X, Saravelos SH, Wang Q, Yanwen X, Li T-C, Zhou C. Endometrial thickness as a predictor of pregnancy outcomes in 10787 fresh IVF–ICSI cycles. Reproductive Biomedicine Online. 2016;**33**:197-205

[25] Wu Y, Gao X, Xiang L, Xi J, Jiang S, Sun Y, et al. Endometrial thickness affects the outcome of in vitro fertilization and embryo transfer in normal responders after GnRH antagonist administration. Reproductive Biology and Endocrinology. 2014;**12**:96

[26] Sher G, Herbert C, Maassarani G, Jacobs MH. Assessment of the late proliferative phase endometrium by ultrasonography in patients undergoing in-vitro fertilization and embryo transfer (TVF/ET). Human Reproduction. 1991;**6**(2):232-237

[27] Zhao J, Zhang Q, Wang Y, Li Y. Endometrial pattern, thickness and growth in predicting pregnancy outcome following 3319 IVF cycle. Reproductive Biomedicine Online. 2014;**29**:291-298

[28] Coelho N, Martins WP, Lima M, Barbosa M, Nastri C, Ferriani R, et al. Ovarian response is a better predictor of clinical pregnancy rate following embryo transfer than is thin endometrium or presence of an endometrioma. Ultrasound in Obstetrics & Gynecology. 2015;**46**:501-505

[29] Shterev A. Ultrasound diagnostics of phase changes in the endometrium. Diagnostic and Therapeutic Ultrasound. 1993;**1**:45-47. in Cyrillic

[30] Zhang T, He Y, Wang Y, Zhu Q, Yang J, Xiaoming ZY, et al. The role of three-dimensional power Doppler ultrasound parameters measured on hCG day in the prediction of pregnancy during in vitro fertilization treatment. European Journal of Obstetrics and Gynecology and Reproductive Biology. 2016;**203**:66-71

[31] Timeva T, Milachich T, St K, At S. Assessment of endometrial characteristics conducive to implantation. Reproductive Health. 2017;**25**:9-13. in Cyrillic

[32] Bozdag G, Aksan G, Esinler I, Yarali H. What is the role of office hysteroscopy in women with failed IVF cycles? Reproductive Biomedicine Online. 2008;**17**:410-415

[33] Fatemi HM, Kasius JC, Timmermans A, van Disseldorp J, Fauser BC, Deveroey P, et al. Prevalence of unsuspected uterine cavity abnormalities diagnosed by office hysteroscopy prior to in vitro fertilization. Human Reproduction. 2010;**25**:1959-1965

[34] Hooker AB, Lemmers M, Thurkow AL, Heymans MW, Opmeer BC, Brölmann HA, et al. Systematic review and meta-analysis of intrauterine adhesions after miscarriage: Prevalence, risk factors and longterm reproductive outcome. Human Reproduction Update. 2014;**20**:2062-2078

[35] Galliano D, Bellver J, Díaz-García C, Simon C, Pellicer A. ART and uterine pathology: How relevant is the maternal side for implantation? Human Reproduction Update. 2015;**21**:13-38

[36] Sarani SA, Ghaffari Novin M, et al. Morfological evidence for the "implantation window" in human luminal endometrium. Human Reproduction. 1999;**14**(12):3101-3106

[37] Buscher U, Schmiady H, et al. Determining implantation time frame of the trophoblast by hCG level monitoring. Geburtshilfe und Frauenheilkunde. 1995;**55**(12):661-665

[38] Klentzeris LD. The role of endometrium in implantation. Human Reproduction. 1997;**12**(11):170-175

[39] Dimitriadis E, White C, Jones R, Salamonsen L. Cytokines, chemokines and growth factors in endometrium related to implantation. Human Reproduction Update. 2005;**11**(6):613-630

[40] Lessey BA. Assessment of endometrial receptivity. Fertility and Sterility. 2011;**96**:522-529

[41] Urman B, Yakin K, Balaban B. Recurrent implantation failure in assisted reproduction: How to counsel and manage. A. General considerations and treatment options that may benefit the couple. Reproductive Biomedicine Online. 2005;**11**(3):371-381

[42] Brandenberger AW, Bersinger NA, Huber PR, et al. CA-125 concentrations in the serum and pregnancy outcome in IVF cycles. Journal of Assisted Reproduction and Genetics. 1998;**15**(6):390-394

[43] Acosta A, Elberger L. Endometrial dating and determination of the implantation windiw in healthy fertile women. Fertility and Sterility. 2000;**73**(4):788-798

[44] Al-Rumaih HM, Price KM, Gillott DJ, Grudzinskas GJ. Proteomic analysis of uterine flushings from infertile women in the proliferative phase of the menstrual cycle with respect to estrogen level. Middle East Fertility Society Journal. 2006;**11**(3):183-190

[45] Berlanga O, Garrido T, Martınez S, Pellicer A, Bradshaw HB, Simo'n C. Lipidomic profiling of endometrial fluid as a noninvasive diagnostic tool of human endometrial receptivity. Fertility and Sterility. 2010;**94**(4):S217

[46] Salamonsen L, Edgell T, Rombauts L, Stephens A, Robertson D, Rainczuk A, et al. Proteomics of the human endometrium and uterine fluid: A pathway to biomarker discovery. Fertility and Sterility. 2013;**99**:1086-1092

[47] Cheong Y, Boomsma C, Heijnen C, Macklon N. Uterine secretomics: A window on the maternal-embryo interface. Fertility and Sterility. 2013;**99**:1093-1099

[48] Vilella F, Ramirez LB, Simón C. Lipidomics as an emerging tool to predict endometrial receptivity. Fertility and Sterility. 2013;**99**:1100-1106

[49] Revel A, Achache H, Stevens J, Smith Y, Reich R. MicroRNAs are associated with human embryo implantation defects. Human Reproduction. 2011;**26**(10):2830-2840

[50] Ali SB, Jeelall Y, Pennell CE, Hart R, McLean-Tooke A, Lucas M. The role of immunological testing and intervention in reproductive medicine: A fertile collaboration? American Journal of Reproductive Immunology. Mar 2018;**79**(3). DOI: 10.1111/aji.12784

[51] Kyurkchiev D, Ivanova-Todorova E, Hayrabedyan S, Altankova I, et al. Female sex steroid hormones modify some regulatory properties of monocyte-derived dendritic cells. American Journal of Reproductive Immunology. 2007;**58**(5):425-433

[52] Macklon N. Factors affecting implantation. In: Abstracts of MSRM Intrnational Meeting "Implantation-Recurrent Miscarriages Science and Clinical Aspects". Chania, Crete: Mediterranean Society for Reproductive Medicine (MSRM); 2010. pp. 14-15

[53] Brosens J, Hodgetts A, Feroze-Zaidi F, Sherwin J, Fusi L, Salker M, et al. Proteomic analysis of endometrium from fertile and infertile patients suggests a role for apolipoprotein A-I in embryo implantation failure and endometriosis. Molecular Human Reproduction. 2010;**16**(4):273-285

[54] Devroey P, Bourgain C, Macklon NS, Fauser BC. Reproductive biology and IVF: Ovarian stimulation and endometrial receptivity. Trends in Endocrinology and Metabolism. 2004;**15**:84-90

[55] Papanikolaou E, Bourgain C, Fatemi H, Verpoest W, Polyzos NP, De Brabanter A, et al. Endometrial advancement after triggering with recombinant or urinary hCG: A randomized controlled pilot study. Reproductive Biomedicine Online. 2010;**21**(1):50-55

[56] Aboulghar M. Stimulation protocols and implantation. In: Abstracts of MSRM Intrnational Meeting "Implantation-Recurrent Miscarriages Science and Clinical Aspects". Chania, Crete:

Mediterranean Society for Reproductive Medicine (MSRM); 2010. p. 19

[57] Haouzi D, Dechaud H, Assou S, De Vos J, Hamamah S. Insights into human endometrial receptivity from transcriptomic and proteomic data. Reproductive Biomedicine Online. 2012;**24**:23-34

[58] Díaz-Gimeno P, Horcajadas JA, Martınez-Conejero JA, Esteban FJ, Alama P, Pellicer A, et al. A genomic diagnostic tool for human endometrial receptivity based on the transcriptomic signature. Fertility and Sterility. 2011;**95**:50-60

[59] Díaz-Gimeno P, Ruiz-Alonso M, Blesa D, Bosch N, Martínez-Conejero JA, Alama P, et al. The accuracy and reproducibility of the endometrial receptivity array is superior to histology as a diagnostic method for endometrial receptivity. Fertility and Sterility. 2013;**99**:508-517

[60] Garrido-Gómez T, Ruiz-Alonso M, Blesa D, Diaz-Gimeno P, Vilella F, Simón C. Profiling the gene signature of endometrial receptivity: Clinical results. Fertility and Sterility. 2013;**99**:1078-1085

[61] Bhagwat S, Chandrashekar D, Kakar R, Davuluri S, Bajpai A, Nayak S, et al. Endometrial receptivity: A revisit to functional genomic studies on human endometrium and creation of HGEx-ERdb. PLoSOne. 2013;**8**(3):e58419. DOI: 10.1371

[62] Koler M, Achache H, Tsfrir A, Smith Y, Revel A, Reich R. Disrupted gene pattern in patients with repeated in vitro fertilization (IVF) failure. Human Reproduction. 2009;**24**:2541-2548

[63] The ESHRE Guideline Group on Female Fertility Preservation, Richard A Anderson, Frédéric Amant, Didi Braat, Arianna D'Angelo, Susana M Chuva de Sousa Lopes, et al. ESHRE guideline: female fertility preservation. Human Reproduction Open. 2020;**2020**(4):hoaa052. DOI: 10.1093/hropen/hoaa052

[64] Liu X, Li W, Wen W, et al. Natural cycle versus hormone replacement therapy as endometrial preparation in ovulatory women undergoing frozen-thawed embryo transfer: The compete open-label randomized controlled trial. PLoS Medicine. 2025;**22**(6):1-18

Chapter 3

The Role of Gynaecological Pathology in Fertility Preservation: Theory and Practical Experience

Constantina Claudia Mateoiu

Abstract

A developing field that straddles the boundaries of gynaecological pathology and reproductive medicine is fertility preservation. Around the world, a large number of women in their prepubertal, postpubescent, and reproductive years receive a cancer diagnosis. Depending on the patient's age and the type of treatment, oncological treatments might impair future fertility in a variety of ways. International associations advise that cancer survivors should not be dissuaded from getting pregnant and that cancer patients should be informed about how cancer treatments affect their reproductive health. The importance of gynaecological pathology in detecting, diagnosing, and treating illnesses, therapies like chemotherapy, and other variables that affect fertility is examined in this chapter. It provides a theoretical synopsis of the pathophysiological processes at play as well as new technologies to inform therapy choices. In order to improve the outcomes for patients dealing with reproductive health issues, the integration of histopathological findings into fertility-sparing strategies is emphasised, along with the value of multidisciplinary collaboration and the critical role pathology plays in individualised fertility preservation.

Keywords: reproductive pathology, organoid, tissue engineering, viability assessment, follicle density, *in vitro* follicle development, multiplexed immunoassays, immunohistochemistry, malignant cell contamination, gene expression arrays, vitrification, slow freezing

1. Introduction

For cancer patients of reproductive age, fertility preservation (FP) consultation is vital in making decisions because it offers vital information and support [1, 2]. Globally, over 2 million women of reproductive age and nearly 9000 women of prepubertal age received cancer diagnoses in 2020 [3]. While breast cancer is the most frequent malignancy among women of childbearing age, lymphoproliferative disorders have the highest prevalence among prepubertal females [3]. A greater rate of survival following cancer has been made possible in recent decades by early diagnosis and improvements in oncological therapy [4]. Surgery [5, 6], radiotherapy [7], and pharmaceutical treatments [8–10] are examples of oncological therapies that can negatively impact the ovarian reserve through a variety of mechanisms, thereby compromising fertility to varying degrees. In order to guarantee these women a high quality of life and the chance to conceive, interest in oncofertility has skyrocketed in the recent decades.

Implementation is still deficient even though guidelines advise having appropriate conversations about FP prior to cancer treatment [11]. To increase cancer patients' knowledge of and access to FP options, a multidisciplinary strategy including oncologists and reproductive specialists is necessary [11, 12]. Only 12% of women remember fertility conversations, indicating that oncologists continue to refer patients at low rates [13].

Personalised consultations, non-directive methods, precise information, and resource connections are the main focusses of current interventions [1]. The ability to ask questions, the timing of consultations, and financial considerations are some of the factors that affect decision-making [2].

The cryopreservation of embryos or oocytes and the cryopreservation and reimplantation of ovarian tissue are voluntary FP methods [14]. For patients who must begin cancer treatment as soon as possible or who are prepubescent, the latter approach is their only choice. Furthermore, ovariopexy is advised in cases of pelvic radiation therapy, and fertility-sparing surgery is considered when feasible [15]. The gonadotropin-releasing hormone agonist (GnRHa) is advised for the preservation of ovarian function if none of the previously listed elective FP procedures can be carried out [16].

The most popular option among patients is embryo cryopreservation, which is followed by ovarian tissue and oocyte cryopreservation [17]. With no discernible variations in live birth rates, clinical pregnancy rates vary from 34.9 to 49.0% across various preservation techniques [18]. However, compared to embryo cryopreservation, ovarian tissue cryopreservation led to a much lower number of miscarriages [18].

Despite these positive results, cancer patients usually generate fewer oocytes than age-matched controls [17]. As survival rates increase, individualised FP techniques are becoming increasingly important for maintaining the quality of life for cancer patients [19].

Although the clinical and laboratory elements of FP are the main emphasis of reproductive medicine, pathology is essential to guaranteeing the efficacy, safety, and viability of stored gametes and gonadal tissues.

2. Histopathological assessment of ovarian tissue

The histopathological effects of cryopreservation techniques on ovarian tissue are quantifiable. Compared to vitrification, slow freezing of the human ovarian cortex often maintains follicle density and form more closely [20]. However, as compared to fresh tissue, both cryopreservation techniques cause some level of cellular stress and alter vascular indicators, mitochondrial activity, and gene expression. Differences in cryoprotectant levels, freezing methods, and specimen characteristics account for the variations observed in the histopathological results.

The effects of ovarian tissue cryopreservation on cellular viability and integrity are not entirely consistent. According to a number of studies, tissue function indicators frequently decrease following thawing, while follicle numbers are generally unaffected [21].

Following tissue transplantation, different people have different reproductive outcomes. While some studies show tissue function for up to 10 years and significant functional recovery (93% endocrine recovery; 58% fertilisation rate), others report that over 90% of patients have low ovarian reserve or premature ovarian failure. Severe problems are still uncommon, with reported pregnancy rates ranging from 18 to 71% and live birth rates from 18 to 41% [22].

2.1 Pre-cryopreservation evaluation of ovarian tissue: Examination of follicle density, stromal integrity, and signs of disease

The viability of post-thaw ovarian tissue and the possibility of fertility restoration are greatly impacted by variations in follicle density and stromal integrity. Within the ovarian cortex, primordial follicle density varies greatly and declines with age [23]. The survival of ovarian tissue may be compromised by cryopreservation and thawing, which can increase follicle degeneration, decrease hormone synthesis, and decrease glucose uptake [21]. Nonetheless, follicle viability, shape, and developmental potential can be preserved using optimised slow freezing methods [24].

Following thawing, vitrification has no effect on tissue morphology and follicle density; nevertheless, following culture shows decreased follicle density and survival [25]. With changes in WNT signalling and hormonal regulatory pathways indicating areas for protocol modification, transcriptomic analysis reveals the slight impacts of vitrification on gene expression [25]. These results emphasise how crucial it is to optimise ovarian tissue preservation for fertility restoration by taking into account factors including follicle density, stromal integrity, and cryopreservation methods.

2.2 Post-thaw analysis and viability assessment: Structural integrity of preserved tissues

Human tissue samples that have been cryopreserved may experience structural alterations and damage that compromise their integrity when they defrost. Research has indicated that distinct freezing and thawing procedures yield differing levels of tissue preservation. Compared to slow freezing, flash freezing and the use of cryopreservation chemicals result in fewer changes to tissue microstructure [26]. Tissue viability and follicle survival were greatly impacted by the protocol selection, underscoring the necessity of a methodical assessment of clinically applied protocols in order to maximise preservation results [27].

Molecular and microscopic methods provide complimentary ways to evaluate tissue viability during freezing and thawing. Cell viability in cryopreserved venous grafts may be assessed using fluorescence vital dyes and confocal imaging; both slow and quick thawing procedures produce initial viability above 70% [28]. Propidium iodide viability assay (PIVA) was found to be more sensitive than trypan blue exclusion (TBE) for identifying dead cells in primordial germ cells [29].

In ovarian tissue, lactate dehydrogenase (LDH) release quantification efficiently assessed cytotoxicity, while trypan blue and calcein AM/ethidium homodimer-1 staining produced results for follicle viability assessment that were comparable [30]. TUNEL-based DNA fragmentation analysis can help assess tissue quality after cryopreservation [30].

2.3 Viability markers for successful transplantation or *in vitro* maturation

In order to improve fertility treatments, viability markers for successful oocyte transplantation or *in vitro* maturation (IVM) are essential. Cumulus cells have been found to contain a number of putative markers, such as HAS2, INHBA, EGFR, and GREM1 [31]. ATP5e and ATP5o may be indicators for oocyte viability following IVM [32], according to RNA-seq research. Follicles, immunocytochemistry, electron microscopy, and endocrine tests are some of the techniques used to assess oocyte growth and survival in culture [33].

Glycolytic activity has been demonstrated to be a valid non-invasive indicator of embryo viability, with mice showing better implantation rates when glycolytic activity is low [34]. The selection of viable oocytes and embryos for transplantation or further development may be greatly enhanced by these indicators, which could also raise the success rates of reproductive therapies and offer important new information on the molecular mechanisms governing oocyte competence.

For assisted reproductive technology (ART) to be successful, oocyte quality must be evaluated and optimised. The validity of conventional morphological assessments of oocytes and embryos is debatable, despite their widespread use [35]. To forecast oocyte competency and embryo quality, scientists are looking at new objective cellular and molecular markers. These comprise extrinsic indicators like follicular cell apoptosis and growth factor levels in follicular fluid, as well as intrinsic variables like mitochondrial state and glucose-6-phosphate dehydrogenase activity [35, 36].

Recent research has examined the apoptosis, transcriptome features, mitochondrial quality, and telomere length of granulosa cells as possible sources of biomarkers [37]. Even while non-invasive molecular diagnostic methods have advanced, a completely accurate and reasonably priced test is still elusive [38]. Nonetheless, gene expression in cumulus cells exhibits potential as a predictor of the quality of embryos and the results of pregnancies [38].

Recent studies have investigated viability markers for oocytes and embryos following cryopreservation and *in vitro* maturation (IVM). Atp5e and Atp5o were found to be promising indicators for oocyte viability following IVM [32] by RNA-seq analysis. According to research, freezing immature oocytes does not produce the same effects as developing them to the MII stage prior to cryopreservation [39]. Numerous techniques, such as follicular counts, immunocytochemistry, and fluorescent viability indicators, have been developed to assess follicle growth and survival in culture [33].

Developmentally competent embryos exhibit decreased metabolic activity [40], and post-thaw amino acid metabolism can predict the blastocyst development with 87% accuracy. The developmental potential of Grade I embryos can be differentiated by metabolic profile, indicating that amino acid turnover may be a useful criterion for choosing cryopreserved embryos for transfer in clinical IVF [40].

The LIVE/DEAD assay has been shown to have a strong predictive value for follicle developmental potential in cryopreserved ovarian tissue, with >85% viability indicating retained potential with regard to cryopreserved reproductive cells [41].

Despite having equal morphometric parameters, fresh *in vitro* maturation (fIVM) of immature oocytes produced higher maturation rates than vitrified-IVM (vIVM) [42]. Trypan blue (TB) staining outperformed calcein AM/ethidium homodimer-1 (CaAM/EthD-1) for assessing the vitality of isolated human follicles in both fresh and thawed samples in terms of reliability and inter-observer agreement [43]. These results emphasise how crucial it is to use the right viability tests for diverse biological products because a number of variables might affect how effective they are [44].

3. Pathological considerations in cancer patients undergoing FP

3.1 Impact of chemotherapy and radiotherapy on ovarian tissues

Premenopausal women with cancer who get high-dose chemotherapy may experience detectable injury to their ovaries. A range of ovarian alterations were caused by combined chemotherapy and radiation therapy, ranging from intact function (59%) with normal hormone levels and ongoing menstruation to severe failure (41% of cases) with missing follicles and decreased volume. In the ovarian cortex, high doses of radiation and chemotherapy can cause a gradual, dose-related loss of primordial follicles [45].

By restarting menstruation, displaying follicular activity on ultrasonography, and reaching normalised hormone levels, autotransplantation of cryopreserved ovarian tissue may restore function. Two embryos are produced after *in vitro* fertilisation. Ovarian volume, antral follicle count, follicle-stimulating hormone, oestradiol, and menstruation are among the markers of ovarian function that are measured.

One study found that 59% of participants had preserved function (normal ovarian volume, presence of antral follicles, normal follicle-stimulating hormone, normal oestradiol, and continued menstruation), whereas 41% had diminished ovarian reserve (low ovarian volume, no antral follicles, and high follicle-stimulating hormone) [45].

In one study, all three autotransplanted women restored ovarian function, with recovery status being reported [46]. According to a different study, ovarian tissue can be safely and effectively collected from cancer patients using laparoscopic ovarian biopsy with a round biopter. The absence of malignant cells in the samples analysed from ovarian cortical tissue from individuals with Hodgkin's disease supports the safety of ovarian tissue cryopreservation in this situation. Nonetheless, each disease should have its risk of malignant cell transmission assessed [45].

The production of two embryos from the cryopreserved tissue following *in vitro* fertilisation indicates that autotransplantation of cryopreserved ovarian tissue can restore ovarian function and that post-transplantation gametogenesis is functional [46].

High-dose chemotherapy is consistently linked to both histological and functional ovarian damage in premenopausal women with cancer, according to the current data. A limited number of examples support the possibility of functional recovery with autotransplantation of cryopreserved tissue.

To guarantee the accurate and repeatable results, quality control and assurance are essential in FP tissue analysis. The integrity of ovarian samples is preserved through standardised procedures for tissue handling, processing, and storage. Accurate diagnosis is ensured by routine validation of molecular assays, imaging systems, and staining methods. Laboratory variability is reduced through internal and external quality control systems, such as blinded reviews and proficiency testing. In FP programmes, consistent QA/QC procedures promote clinical decision-making and protect patient safety.

3.2 Detection of malignant cells in ovarian biopsies

Multiplexed immunoassays (including bead-based technologies), immunohistochemistry, recursive descent partition analysis, gene expression arrays, and reverse transcription polymerase chain reaction are methods for identifying malignant cells in ovarian biopsies.

The most effective approach for directly identifying malignant cells in ovarian tissue samples is immunohistochemistry using well-selected marker panels, according to data from several investigations. When used on ovarian tissue, immunohistochemistry provides the best proof for detecting cancerous cells in biopsies. About 99.4% of tumours were found using a panel of claudin-3, cancer antigen 125, and mucin 1, and this number rose to 100% when vascular endothelial growth factor was included [47]. Immunohistochemistry strengthens the usefulness of histotypes for tissue-based diagnosis by increasing their repeatability [48].

Studies utilising molecular methods, such as reverse transcription polymerase chain reaction and gene expression arrays, on the other hand, found potential biomarkers but did not specifically disclose clinical diagnostic performance in biopsies. Similarly, serum-based multiplex immunoassays [49, 50], which were not directly validated in tissue biopsies, achieved respectable sensitivity and specificity with panels that included human epididymis protein 4, C-reactive protein, cancer antigen 125, and epidermal growth factor receptor. However, these results apply to blood samples rather than ovarian biopsies. Multiplexed immunoassay was reported to have an 82.3% detection rate. Using reverse transcription polymerase chain reaction and immunohistochemistry, a number of elevated genes (NOTCH3, E2F3, RACGAP1, and HN1) have been recognised as putative molecular markers [47].

In all investigations, higher reported diagnostic accuracy was linked to the use of marker panels as opposed to single markers. About 99.4% of ovarian tumours could be detected in tissue samples thanks to the methodical selection and validation of marker combinations (claudin-3, cancer antigen 125, mucin 1, and vascular endothelial growth factor) [47]. In the study sample, detection reached 100% when vascular endothelial growth factor was added. Serum biomarker combinations (e.g., C-reactive protein, cancer antigen 125, and epidermal growth factor receptor) performed better than individual markers [49, 50]. Cancer antigen 125 is still a key biomarker, but when combined with additional indicators, it significantly improved diagnosis accuracy. Although useful for finding biomarkers, serum-based research might not be entirely equivalent to tissue-based diagnostic precision.

In summary, studies have demonstrated that immunohistochemistry, especially when combined with specialised marker panels, is the most successful diagnostic method for detecting malignant cells in ovarian biopsies.

3.3 Ensuring the safety of preserved tissue use in cancer survivors

The degree of malignant cell contamination in cryopreserved ovarian tissue varies according to the cancer type and the method of detection. When it comes to tissue preservation, some safety factors need to be taken into account. Preoperative imaging in pre-preservation screening can stop tissue with obvious disease from being collected and stored, as shown in the included research on haematological malignancies. Sensitive molecular testing, including RT-PCR for illness-specific markers, was essential for post-preservation testing in the included investigations in order to identify minimum residual disease before reimplantation. Due to the possibility of reintroducing cancer, the included studies advise against autotransplantation when it comes to reimplantation regimens for leukaemia and other high-risk malignancies. Autotransplantation may be an option for low-risk tumours (such lymphoma and low-stage breast cancer), but only after extensive testing and screening.

Molecular tests (e.g., RT-PCR) and xenotransplantation can identify malignant cells in as many as 50% of samples in leukaemia (acute lymphoblastic and chronic myeloid) and Ewing sarcoma; for instance, one study revealed that 2 out of 6 cases of chronic myeloid leukaemia and 7 out of 10 cases of acute lymphoblastic leukaemia were positive. On the other hand, specimens of lymphoma and low-stage breast cancer tissue produce negative histology and immunohistochemistry results. Sensitive molecular screening and preoperative imaging were demonstrated to help rule out overt disease, and one haematologic investigation found a 1.7% positive rate by real-time RT-PCR [51].

A risk-stratified approach describes how tissue preservation techniques affect recontamination risk in a way that corresponds with the cancer type and the sensitivity of post-preservation testing methods: low risk with lymphoma and low-stage breast cancer, where the results support consideration of autotransplantation when thorough screening protocols are followed [52, 53]; uncertain/variable risk with colorectal, gastric, endometrial, and cervical cancers [52]; and high risk with leukaemia and Ewing sarcoma, in which autotransplantation is contraindicated [51].

For leukaemia, lymphoma, and breast cancer, the quality of the evidence is regarded as moderate. For Ewing sarcoma, the evidence quality is categorised as low. The evidence regarding other solid tumours is typically weak or requires a case-by-case assessment.

Histology, immunohistochemistry, molecular techniques (PCR or RT-PCR), xenografting, and preoperative imaging are employed as the detection methods.

Histology alone was unable to identify malignant contamination in a number of the included trials when molecular techniques yielded positive results, suggesting poor sensitivity [51]. Histology and immunohistochemistry did not find any contamination in breast cancer, although there is still some doubt because molecular testing was not done [53].

When histology was negative, malignant cells were found using quantitative reverse transcription polymerase chain reaction (RT-PCR) and real-time RT-PCR, especially in leukaemia and chronic myeloid leukaemia. In the included trials, PCR-based techniques that targeted illness-specific markers (such T-cell receptor/immunoglobulin clones and BCR-ABL) were crucial for the sensitive detection of minimal residual disease [51].

The vitality and carcinogenic potential of malignant cells in ovarian tissue from leukaemia patients were verified by xenografting to immunocompromised mice. Although xenotransplantation is not commonly utilised in clinical practice, the included systematic review demonstrates its value as a confirmatory technique [52].

In summary, histology alone is not a suitable detection approach. For a thorough safety evaluation, particularly in high-risk populations, molecular and functional tests (such RT-PCR and xenotransplantation) are required.

Regarding ovarian tissue contamination, it should be noted that molecular techniques [51, 52, 54] were used to detect it, but histology and immunohistochemistry were not used in any investigation. There has been no description of contamination found in cases of lymphoma or breast cancer.

Autotransplantation in leukaemia survivors was not advised due to contamination found in leukaemia or Ewing sarcoma [52]. Preoperative imaging and sensitive molecular diagnostics before transplantation are preferable [54]. Autotransplantation is safe in this group, as there was no evidence of contamination in low-stage breast cancer; nonetheless, additional research is necessary [53].

Since recontamination risks differ depending on the type of cancer and need to be confirmed using suitable detection tools, tissue preservation procedures necessitate cancer-specific treatments.

To reduce the risk of cancer recurrence after ovarian tissue autotransplantation, a multimodal approach to safety is required, including preoperative imaging, molecular testing, and, when practical, functional assays. Small sample sizes, a lack of standardised procedures, and insufficient reporting of participant and preservation characteristics constrain the strength of the evidence basis in the included studies.

Coordination of patient care, particularly when it comes to cancer patients' FP, depends on efficient ways to communicate between pathologists, reproductive endocrinologists, and oncologists. Oncologists use the comprehensive diagnostic and prognostic data that pathologists provide regarding tumours to decide on treatment plans. Effective communication between pathologists, reproductive endocrinologists, and oncologists is essential for patient care coordination, especially when it comes to preserving fertility in cancer patients. Pathologists give oncologists detailed diagnostic and prognostic information about tumours, which oncologists utilise to determine therapy strategies.

4. Emerging technologies in reproductive pathology

4.1 Use of modern diagnostic techniques to identify viable follicles

The main outcome measures evaluated in reproductive pathology are typically follicle vitality, follicle count, and follicle presence or identification. AMH expression in follicles, serum AMH levels, and metastatic detection were further results.

Serum Anti-Müllerian Hormone (AMH) measurement, glucose uptake, neutral red staining, Haematoxylin and Eosin (H&E) histology, immunohistochemistry, Full-Field Optical Coherence Tomography (FF-OCT) imaging, ultrasound, semi-automated image analysis, Proliferating Cell Nuclear Antigen (PCNA) immunohistochemistry, LIVE/DEAD fluorescence assay, and xenotransplantation in Severe Combined Immunodeficiency (SCID) mice were among the detection techniques. The main resource needs for each approach vary. Since each approach depends on different resources, it is difficult to compare them directly or use them interchangeably.

The reference standard is haematoxylin and eosin (H&E) histology, which has been found to have intermediate accuracy and observer variability. Biopsy/histopathology and comparison with other techniques are used for validation [55]. It requires a typical histology lab and takes a moderately lengthy time to process.

The use of PCNA immunohistochemistry, which reports better accuracy and consistency than H&E and less observer variability with automation, is employed. In contrast to hand counts, semi-automated image analysis is used for validation [55]. Microscopy or image analysis software, immunostaining reagents, and training (semi-automated PCNA analysis) are required, and the processing time is moderate.

The use of blood AMH and anti-Müllerian hormone (AMH) immunostaining demonstrates a moderate predictive value (66.7% for positive and 60% for negative) as well as an association with the presence of follicles. Histology is used for validation, but it proved insufficient as a stand-alone marker [56]. Enzyme-Linked

Immunosorbent Assay (ELISA) kits and immunostaining reagents are needed, and processing time is brief.

The use of the LIVE/DEAD fluorescent assay has been shown to have higher sensitivity than histology post-xenotransplant and high viability detection (87.1 ± 3.5%). Comparison with histology following xenotransplantation [41] served as validation. It requires dyes and fluorescence microscopy and has a quick processing time.

High-resolution, quick, and noninvasive Full-Field Optical Coherence Tomography (FF-OCT) imaging is utilised to detect metastases and follicles without sacrificing viability. Validation is done by comparing viability assays and H&E histopathology [57]. It takes only a few minutes to process, although sterile conditions and an FF-OCT instrument are needed.

In AMH, LIVE/DEAD, quantitative accuracy (also known as percentage viability or Positive Predictive Value/Negative Predictive Value) is typically reported. For H&E and PCNA immunohistochemistry, observer variability is frequently studied, and for PCNA immunohistochemistry and semi-automated image analysis, automation or semi-automation is explored. Every technique, with the exception of H&E, is verified by comparison with histology or other accepted techniques.

Every technique has some technical limitations; none are completely free of them. A few of these restrictions are especially significant and deserve further investigation. The main technical difficulties with the methods are highlighted by the following points:

- Haematoxylin and eosin (H&E) histology and Proliferating Cell Nuclear Antigen (PCNA) immunohistochemistry observer variability.
- Haematoxylin and eosin (H&E) histology involves a laborious procedure and destructive analysis.
- The need for antibodies for immunohistochemistry of the Proliferating Cell Nuclear Antigen (PCNA).
- Digital infrastructure and configuration are necessary for semi-automated PCNA analysis.
- Moderate predictive value for Anti-Müllerian Hormone (AMH) immunostaining/serum (not enough on its own).
- The LIVE/DEAD fluorescence assay's viability and specialised equipment requirements were overestimated.
- The imaging technique known as Full-Field Optical Coherence Tomography (FF-OCT) is expensive and scarce, and requires technical mastery.

The definition of viability varies from study to study. Viability necessitated an intact oocyte and more than 50% of granulosa cells to be alive [41]; a LIVE/DEAD assay result of >85% indicated retained embryonic potential. After Full-Field Optical Coherence Tomography (FF-OCT) imaging, there was no discernible decrease in viability as measured by glucose uptake and neutral red staining [57]. Anti-Müllerian Hormone (AMH) levels and follicle presence serve as stand-ins for viability [56]. Instead of emphasising direct viability, another study concentrated on follicle count [55].

When identifying viable ovarian follicles, immunohistochemistry and molecular diagnostics produce results that are different from those obtained using conventional haematoxylin and eosin (H&E) histology. Research using H&E as a reference [41, 56, 57] reported delayed processing and the modest accuracy with significant observer variability. On the other hand, compared to manual H&E counts, one study found that proliferating cell nuclear antigen (PCNA) immunohistochemistry [55] increased accuracy and decreased observer bias, particularly when combined with semi-automated image processing. Follicle presence was reported to have a positive predictive value of 66.7% and a negative predictive value of 60% in one study that used anti-Müllerian hormone (AMH) immunostaining [56]. Another investigation that used a LIVE/DEAD fluorescence assay found that the viability rate was 87.1 ± 3.5%, which was higher than the conventional histological evaluation after xenotransplantation [41]. A proof-of-concept research using Full-Field Optical Coherence Tomography (FF-OCT) imaging showed that follicles could be found quickly and noninvasively without sacrificing tissue viability [57].

This section concludes with an integrative analysis that synthesises the main conclusions to offer a thorough comprehension of the findings:

- When detecting viable ovarian follicles, immunohistochemistry (Proliferating Cell Nuclear Antigen, Anti-Müllerian Hormone) and molecular diagnostics (LIVE/DEAD, Anti-Müllerian Hormone) offer more accuracy and/or consistency than conventional histology techniques.

- Semi-automated image processing further improved reproducibility and decreased observer bias.

- Full-Field Optical Coherence Tomography (FF-OCT) is a noninvasive imaging technique that allows for quick evaluation while maintaining tissue viability.

- Small sample sizes, inconsistent viability criteria, and a lack of standardised sensitivity/specificity reporting typically limit the methodology description.

- The generalisability of these findings is limited by the use of animal models, the emphasis on particular clinical populations (such as cancer or premature ovarian failure), and the lack of long-term functional outcome data.

- Although there was a tendency towards noninvasive, automated, and objective approaches, each approach had at least one technical drawback.

In respect to accurately determining viable ovarian follicles, modern diagnostic methods such as PCNA immunohistochemistry and LIVE/DEAD fluorescence perform better than conventional H&E histology while lowering processing time and observer bias.

4.2 Organoid and tissue engineering approaches for *in vitro* follicle development

Because organoid-based follicle formation procedures imitate the ovarian milieu and lower the danger of malignant cell reintroduction, they may provide a solution to cancer patients' FP issues. Female cancer patients at high risk of infertility from gonadotoxic treatments are the main target population in all of the research, especially those for whom standard ovarian tissue transplantation is contraindicated because of the possibility of malignant cell reintroduction. Based on preclinical and review-level data, the findings of studies describing enhanced *in vitro* follicle formation methods based on organoids for cancer patients' reproductive preservation are encouraging.

According to the studies, the technical methods discussed—which range from organoids and three-dimensional scaffolds to organ-on-a-chip and microfluidic systems—offer benefits in simulating the ovarian milieu and lowering the danger of reintroducing malignant cells.

The rapid evolution of *in vitro* follicle development systems has been demonstrated by current organoid-based technologies. These include three-dimensional scaffolds, decellularized ovarian tissue, and organoid technology that mimics the ovarian microenvironment to support follicle growth and maturation [58, 59]. Additionally, stem cell-derived neo-folliculogenesis and artificial ovary construction are novel approaches, as are organ-on-a-chip and microfluidic platforms, which offer dynamic, biomimetic settings that closely mimic *in vivo* ovarian physiology [59, 60].

Oocyte quality improved simultaneously with 62% follicle growth complete and 8–20% of oocytes reaching metaphase II, according to a study that describes three-dimensional scaffold and pluripotent stem cell induction techniques [58]. Although two-dimensional systems have technical issues with oocyte maturation, another study showed that organ-on-a-chip systems allow metaphase II spindle development and produce up to 90% follicle survival [59]. According to their preclinical models, both research report encouraging preclinical results, including high follicle survival rates (up to 90% in some systems) and indications of oocyte maturation (metaphase II spindle formation). They point out that oocytes' functional competence (such as their capacity for fertilisation) is still being determined and that maturation rates are still below ideal.

Another study presents stem cell-derived neo-folliculogenesis and artificial ovary structures as novel approaches. The use of three-dimensional scaffolds, decellularized ovarian tissue, and organoid technology to mimic the ovarian microenvironment and support follicle growth and maturation has also been described as a technical approach, as have neo-folliculogenesis [60], artificial ovary (including artificial matrix) approaches, and multistage *in vitro* culture [58]. Other approaches include hydrogel encapsulation, extracellular matrix biomaterials [59], and biomimetic models.

According to the included research, the main worry with traditional ovarian tissue transplantation is the danger of reintroducing malignant cells, which makes *in vitro* and organoid-based treatments especially appealing for cancer patients.

The following should be included in the list of benefits of organoid-based technologies: the capacity to replicate biomimetic physiological circumstances or the natural ovarian microenvironment; enhancement of oocyte maturation, folliculogenesis, and overall follicular viability; potential use in clinical settings for regenerative medicine or functional tissue reconstruction; lower risk of malignant cell reintroduction in comparison with autologous ovarian tissue transplantation; utilisation of extracellular matrix (ECM)-based biomaterials and customizable scaffolds to support three-dimensional tissue architecture.

Though they currently have a number of drawbacks, organoid-based technologies present encouraging opportunities for reproductive tissue engineering. These include issues with safety, viability, and scalability; low rates of oocyte maturation and competence; and technical difficulties that call for additional Optimisation. Furthermore, the area is still in its infancy, with little quantitative evidence and unproven therapeutic effectiveness.

Various methods for preserving and restoring fertility are chosen according to the clinical circumstances of each patient. Organoid-based approaches, *in vitro* follicle growth (IVG), artificial ovaries, and organ-on-a-chip systems are preferred for cancer patients, especially those who are at high risk of metastatic disease, because they may reduce the risk of reintroducing malignant cells. Nevertheless, these techniques still have technical limitations, and their effectiveness is still unknown. Although these technologies need more development and confirmation, stem cell-derived follicles and *in vitro* folliculogenesis are seen as promising substitutes in prepubertal females because they do not require tissue transplantation. Both traditional and cutting-edge *in vitro* culture technologies are appropriate for people with general, non-oncological infertility; they provide a lower risk profile, more options, and the possibility of improved oocyte yield and quality.

Research indicates that by achieving 62% follicle growth completeness and reducing the risk of cancer cell reintroduction, organoid-based follicle development methods can help cancer patients maintain their fertility [60]. Combining organoid-based techniques may help high-risk cancer patients maintain their fertility while also drawing attention to technical problems that must be fixed prior to clinical application, including safety concerns, insufficient oocyte maturation, and technological complexity. Oncofertility programmes could include these tactics, particularly for cancer patients who are unable to undergo standard procedures.

By guaranteeing tissue authenticity, quality, and reproducibility, pathologists play a crucial role in the development, characterisation, and validation of organoids for FP. Using their knowledge of tissue architecture and histology, they contribute to the development of uniform standards for organoid morphology, viability, and maturation. Additionally, pathologists use molecular characterisation and immunohistochemistry to verify that organoids accurately mimic natural reproductive tissues.

They help establish standards for safety, functionality, and the lack of cancerous contamination during validation. All things considered, their participation guarantees that organoid models are practically and scientifically reliable for use in future fertility applications.

5. Conclusions

To achieve more accurate prediction of reproductive potential, future pathological research in fertility preservation must prioritise robust and reproducible assessment of tissue viability. Advances in molecular profiling, single-cell technologies, and high-resolution imaging offer unprecedented opportunities to elucidate follicular dynamics and germ cell integrity at an individual-cell level. Moreover, the establishment of standardised, validated biomarkers and harmonised imaging protocols will be essential to improve the accuracy, comparability, and clinical reliability of fertility preservation outcomes across centres, ultimately facilitating broader clinical implementation and personalised patient management.

Author details

Constantina Claudia Mateoiu
Sahlgrenska University Hospital, Gothenburg, Sweden

*Address all correspondence to: claudiamateoiu@gmail.com

References

[1] Han J, Park S, Kim SH. Supporting decision-making regarding fertility preservation in patients with cancer: An integrative review. European Journal of Cancer Care (Engl). 2022;**31**(6):e13748. DOI: 10.1111/ecc.13748. Epub 2022 Oct 24

[2] Kim J, Deal AM, Balthazar U, Kondapalli LA, Gracia C, Mersereau JE. Fertility preservation consultation for women with cancer: Are we helping patients make high-quality decisions? Reproduction Biomedical Online. 2013;**27**(1):96-103. DOI: 10.1016/j.rbmo.2013.03.004. Epub 2013 Mar 26

[3] World Health Organization. International Agency for Research on Cancer. Global Cancer Observatory; 2019. Available from: https://gco.iarc.fr/ [Accessed: 12 May 2022]

[4] Siegel RL, Miller KD, Fuchs HE, Jemal A. Cancer statistics, 2021. CA: A Cancer Journal for Clinicians. 2021;**71**(1):7-33. DOI: 10.3322/caac.21654. Epub 2021 Jan 12. Erratum in: CA Cancer J Clin. 2021;71(4):359. DOI: 10.3322/caac.21669

[5] Gwacham NI, McKenzie ND, Fitzgerald ER, Ahmad S, Holloway RW. Neoadjuvant chemotherapy followed by fertility sparing surgery in cervical cancers size 2-4 cm; emerging data and future perspectives. Gynecologic Oncology. 2021;**162**(3):809-815. DOI: 10.1016/j.ygyno.2021.06.006. Epub 2021 Jun 12

[6] Jiang X, Yang J, Yu M, Xie W, Cao D, Wu M, et al. Oncofertility in patients with stage I epithelial ovarian cancer: Fertility-sparing surgery in young women of reproductive age. World Journal of Surgical Oncology. 2017;**15**(1):154. DOI: 10.1186/s12957-017-1222-4

[7] Hudson MM. Reproductive outcomes for survivors of childhood cancer. Obstetrics and Gynecology. 2010;**116**(5):1171-1183. DOI: 10.1097/AOG.0b013e3181f87c4b

[8] Codacci-Pisanelli G, Del Pup L, Del Grande M, Peccatori FA. Mechanisms of chemotherapy-induced ovarian damage in breast cancer patients. Critical Reviews in Oncology/Hematology. 2017;**113**:90-96. DOI: 10.1016/j.critrevonc.2017.03.009. Epub 2017 Mar 16

[9] Bedoschi G, Navarro PA, Oktay K. Chemotherapy-induced damage to ovary: Mechanisms and clinical impact. Future Oncology. 2016;**12**(20):2333-2344. DOI: 10.2217/fon-2016-0176. Epub 2016 Jul 12

[10] Sella T, Poorvu PD, Ruddy KJ, Gelber SI, Tamimi RM, Peppercorn JM, et al. Impact of fertility concerns on endocrine therapy decisions in young breast cancer survivors. Cancer. 2021;**127**(16):2888-2894. DOI: 10.1002/cncr.33596. Epub 2021 Apr 22

[11] Mahajan N. Fertility preservation in female cancer patients: An overview. Journal of Human Reproductive Sciences. 2015;**8**(1):3-13. DOI: 10.4103/0974-1208.153119

[12] Noyes N, Knopman JM, Melzer K, Fino ME, Friedman B, Westphal LM. Oocyte cryopreservation as a fertility preservation measure for cancer patients. Reproduction Biomedical Online. 2011;**23**(3):323-333. DOI: 10.1016/j.rbmo.2010.11.011. Epub 2010 Nov 24

[13] Hoffman A, Crocker L, Mathur A, Holman D, Weston J, Campbell S, et al.

Patients' and providers' needs and preferences when considering fertility preservation before cancer treatment: Decision-making needs assessment. The Journal of Medical Internet Research Formative Research. 2021;**5**(6):e25083. DOI: 10.2196/25083

[14] Practice Committee of the American Society for Reproductive Medicine. Fertility preservation in patients undergoing gonadotoxic therapy or gonadectomy: A committee opinion. Fertility and Sterility. 2019;**112**(6):1022-1033. DOI: 10.1016/j.fertnstert.2019.09.013

[15] Findeklee S, Radosa JC, Takacs Z, Hamza A, Sima R, Solomayer E, et al. Fertility preservation in female cancer patients: Current knowledge and future perspectives. Minerva Ginecologica. 2019;**71**(4):298-305. DOI: 10.23736/S0026-4784.19.04387-9. Epub 2019 Apr 15

[16] Oktay K, Harvey BE, Partridge AH, Quinn GP, Reinecke J, Taylor HS, et al. Fertility preservation in patients with cancer: ASCO clinical practice guideline update. Journal of Clinical Oncology. 2018;**36**(19):1994-2001. DOI: 10.1200/JCO.2018.78.1914. Epub 2018 Apr 5

[17] Klock SC, Zhang JX, Kazer RR. Fertility preservation for female cancer patients: Early clinical experience. Fertility and Sterility. 2010;**94**(1):149-155. DOI: 10.1016/j.fertnstert.2009.03.028. Epub 2009 May 5

[18] Ní Dhonnabháin B, Elfaki N, Fraser K, Petrie A, Jones BP, Saso S, et al. A comparison of fertility preservation outcomes in patients who froze oocytes, embryos, or ovarian tissue for medically indicated circumstances: A systematic review and meta-analysis. Fertility and Sterility. 2022;**117**(6):1266-1276. DOI: 10.1016/j.fertnstert.2022.03.004. Epub 2022 Apr 19

[19] Chung K, Donnez J, Ginsburg E, Meirow D. Emergency IVF versus ovarian tissue cryopreservation: Decision making in fertility preservation for female cancer patients. Fertility and Sterility. 2013;**99**(6):1534-1542. DOI: 10.1016/j.fertnstert.2012.11.057. Epub 2013 Mar 18

[20] Fabbri R, Vicenti R, Macciocca M, Martino NA, Dell'Aquila ME, Pasquinelli G, et al. Morphological, ultrastructural and functional imaging of frozen/thawed and vitrified/warmed human ovarian tissue retrieved from oncological patients. Human Reproduction. 2016;**31**(8):1838-1849. DOI: 10.1093/humrep/dew134. Epub 2016 Jun 9

[21] Bastings L, Liebenthron J, Westphal JR, Beerendonk CC, van der Ven H, Meinecke B, et al. Efficacy of ovarian tissue cryopreservation in a major European center. Journal Assisted Reproduction Genetics. 2014;**31**(8):1003-1012. DOI: 10.1007/s10815-014-0239-7. Epub 2014 Jun 14

[22] Meirow D, Ra'anani H, Shapira M, Brenghausen M, Derech Chaim S, Aviel-Ronen S, et al. Transplantations of frozen-thawed ovarian tissue demonstrate high reproductive performance and the need to revise restrictive criteria. Fertility and Sterility. 2016;**106**(2):467-474. DOI: 10.1016/j.fertnstert.2016.04.031. Epub 2016 May 12

[23] Schmidt KL, Byskov AG, Nyboe Andersen A, Müller J, Yding Andersen C. Density and distribution of primordial follicles in single pieces of cortex from 21 patients and in individual pieces of cortex from three entire human ovaries. Human Reproduction. 2003;**18**(6):1158-1164. DOI: 10.1093/humrep/deg246

[24] Sanfilippo S, Canis M, Romero S, Sion B, Déchelotte P, Pouly JL, et al.

Quality and functionality of human ovarian tissue after cryopreservation using an original slow freezing procedure. Journal Assisted Reproduction Genetics. 2013;**30**(1):25-34. DOI: 10.1007/s10815-012-9917-5. Epub 2012 Dec 22

[25] Deligiannis SP, Kask K, Modhukur V, Boskovic N, Ivask M, Jaakma Ü, et al. Investigating the impact of vitrification on bovine ovarian tissue morphology, follicle survival, and transcriptomic signature. Journal Assisted Reproduction Genetics. 2024;**41**(4):1035-1055. DOI: 10.1007/s10815-024-03038-4. Epub 2024 Feb 15

[26] Kropatsch K, Daigle N, Duan S, Sontz R, Merchant JL, Sawyer TW. Evaluating the impact of freeze-thaw protocols on tissue microstructural imaging features measured using optical coherence tomography. Proc SPIE 12854. 2024. DOI: 10.1117/12.3001355

[27] Bastings L, Westphal JR, Beerendonk CC, Bekkers RL, Zusterzeel PL, Hendriks JC, et al. Clinically applied procedures for human ovarian tissue cryopreservation result in different levels of efficacy and efficiency. Journal Assisted Reproduction Genetics. 2016;**33**(12):1605-1614. DOI: 10.1007/s10815-016-0816-z. Epub 2016 Oct 6

[28] Mericka P, Janoušek L, Benda A, Lainková R, Sabó J, Dalecká M, et al. Cell viability assessment using fluorescence vital dyes and confocal microscopy in evaluating freezing and thawing protocols used in cryopreservation of allogeneic venous grafts. International Journal Molecular Science. 2021;**22**(19):10653. DOI: 10.3390/ijms221910653

[29] Svoradová A, Makarevich A, Vašíček J, Olexiková L, Dragin S, Chrenek P. Microscopic assessment of dead cell ratio in cryopreserved chicken primordial germ cells. Microscopy and Microanalysis. 2019;**25**(5):1257-1262. DOI: 10.1017/S1431927619014934

[30] Merdassi G, Mazoyer C, Guerin JF, Saad A, Salle B, Lornage J. Examination of viability and quality of ovarian tissue after cryopreservation using simple laboratory methods in ewe. Reproductive Biology and Endocrinololgy. 2011;**9**:78. DOI: 10.1186/1477-7827-9-78

[31] Assidi M, Dufort I, Ali A, Hamel M, Algriany O, Dielemann S, et al. Identification of potential markers of oocyte competence expressed in bovine cumulus cells matured with follicle-stimulating hormone and/or phorbol myristate acetate in vitro. Biololgy of Reproduction. 2008;**79**(2):209-222. DOI: 10.1095/biolreprod.108.067686. Epub 2008 Apr 16

[32] Gao L, Jia G, Li A, Ma H, Huang Z, Zhu S, et al. RNA-Seq transcriptome profiling of mouse oocytes after in vitro maturation and/or vitrification. Science of Reproduction. 2017;**7**(1):13245. DOI: 10.1038/s41598-017-13381-5

[33] Abir R, Nitke S, Ben-Haroush A, Fisch B. In vitro maturation of human primordial ovarian follicles: Clinical significance, progress in mammals, and methods for growth evaluation. Histology and Histopathology. 2006;**21**(8):887-898. DOI: 10.14670/HH-21.887

[34] Lane M, Gardner DK. Selection of viable mouse blastocysts prior to transfer using a metabolic criterion. Human Reproduction. 1996;**11**(9):1975-1978. DOI: 10.1093/oxfordjournals.humrep.a019527

[35] Wang Q, Sun QY. Evaluation of oocyte quality: Morphological, cellular

and molecular predictors. Reproduction Fertility Development. 2007;**19**(1):1-12. DOI: 10.1071/rd06103

[36] Combelles CM, Racowsky C. Assessment and optimization of oocyte quality during assisted reproductive technology treatment. Seminars in Reproductive Medicine. 2005;**23**(3):277-284. DOI: 10.1055/s-2005-872456

[37] Huang R, Zhou W, Zhu Y. Granulosa cell biomarkers to predict oocyte and embryo quality in assisted reproductive technology. Reproductive and Developmental Medicine. 2021;**05**(01):30-37. DOI: 10.4103/2096-2924.313684

[38] Hillier SG. Molecular diagnosis in the ART laboratory: Making it matter. Molecular Human Reproduction. 2010;**16**(8):511-512. DOI: 10.1093/molehr/gaq050. Epub 2010 Jul 7

[39] Lee JA, Barritt J, Moschini RM, Slifkin RE, Copperman AB. Optimizing human oocyte cryopreservation for fertility preservation patients: Should we mature then freeze or freeze then mature? Fertility and Sterility. 2013;**99**(5):1356-1362. DOI: 10.1016/j.fertnstert.2012.11.042. Epub 2012 Dec 21

[40] Stokes PJ, Hawkhead JA, Fawthrop RK, Picton HM, Sharma V, Leese HJ, et al. Metabolism of human embryos following cryopreservation: Implications for the safety and selection of embryos for transfer in clinical IVF. Human Reproduction. 2007;**22**(3):829-835. DOI: 10.1093/humrep/del447. Epub 2006 Nov 30. Erratum in: Hum Reprod. 2007 Apr;22(4):1196

[41] Maltaris T, Kaya H, Hoffmann I, Mueller A, Beckmann MW, Dittrich R. Comparison of xenografting in SCID mice and LIVE/DEAD assay as a predictor of the developmental potential of cryopreserved ovarian tissue. In Vivo. 2006;**20**(1):11-16

[42] Nazari S, Khalili MA, Esmaielzadeh F, Mohsenzadeh M. Maturation capacity, morphology and morphometric assessment of human immature oocytes after vitrification and in-vitro maturation. Iran Journal Reproduction Medicine. 2011;**9**(3):209-216

[43] Sanfilippo S, Canis M, Ouchchane L, Botchorishvili R, Artonne C, Janny L, et al. Viability assessment of fresh and frozen/thawed isolated human follicles: Reliability of two methods (Trypan blue and Calcein AM/ethidium homodimer-1). Journal Assisted Reproduction Genetics. 2011;**28**(12):1151-1156. DOI: 10.1007/s10815-011-9649-y. Epub 2011 Oct 27

[44] Cai Y, Prochazkova M, Kim YS, Jiang C, Ma J, Moses L, et al. Assessment and comparison of viability assays for cellular products. Cytotherapy. 2024;**26**(2):201-209. DOI: 10.1016/j.jcyt.2023.11.008. Epub 2023 Dec 11

[45] Meirow D. Ovarian injury and modern options to preserve fertility in female cancer patients treated with high dose radio-chemotherapy for hemato-oncological neoplasias and other cancers. Leukemia Lymphoma. 1999;**33**(1-2):65-76. DOI: 10.3109/10428199909093726

[46] Schmidt KL, Andersen CY, Loft A, Byskov AG, Ernst E, Andersen AN. Follow-up of ovarian function post-chemotherapy following ovarian cryopreservation and transplantation. Human Reproduction. 2005;**20**(12):3539-3546. DOI: 10.1093/humrep/dei250. Epub 2005 Aug 19

[47] Lu KH, Patterson AP, Wang L, Marquez RT, Atkinson EN, Baggerly KA, et al. Selection of potential markers

for epithelial ovarian cancer with gene expression arrays and recursive descent partition analysis. Clincal Cancer Research. 2004;**10**(10):3291-3300. DOI: 10.1158/1078-0432.CCR-03-0409

[48] Köbel M, Bak J, Bertelsen BI, Carpen O, Grove A, Hansen ES, et al. Ovarian carcinoma histotype determination is highly reproducible, and is improved through the use of immunohistochemistry. Histopathology. 2014;**64**(7):1004-1013. DOI: 10.1111/his.12349. Epub 2014 Mar 7

[49] Bertenshaw GP, Yip P, Seshaiah P, Zhao J, Chen TH, Wiggins WS, et al. Multianalyte profiling of serum antigens and autoimmune and infectious disease molecules to identify biomarkers dysregulated in epithelial ovarian cancer. Cancer Epidemiology, Biomarkers & Prevention. 2008;**17**(10):2872-2881. DOI: 10.1158/1055-9965.EPI-08-0464

[50] Nolen B, Marrangoni A, Velikokhatnaya L, Prosser D, Winans M, Gorelik E, et al. A serum based analysis of ovarian epithelial tumorigenesis. Gynecologic Oncology. 2009;**112**(1):47-54. DOI: 10.1016/j.ygyno.2008.09.043. Epub 2008 Nov 12

[51] Dolmans MM, Marinescu C, Saussoy P, Van Langendonckt A, Amorim C, Donnez J. Reimplantation of cryopreserved ovarian tissue from patients with acute lymphoblastic leukemia is potentially unsafe. Blood. 2010;**116**(16):2908-2914. DOI: 10.1182/blood-2010-01-265751. Epub 2010 Jul 1

[52] Bastings L, Beerendonk CC, Westphal JR, Massuger LF, Kaal SE, van Leeuwen FE, et al. Autotransplantation of cryopreserved ovarian tissue in cancer survivors and the risk of reintroducing malignancy: A systematic review. Human Reproduction Update. 2013;**19**(5):483-506. DOI: 10.1093/humupd/dmt020. Epub 2013 Jun 30

[53] Rosendahl M, Timmermans Wielenga V, Nedergaard L, Kristensen SG, Ernst E, Rasmussen PE, et al. Cryopreservation of ovarian tissue for fertility preservation: No evidence of malignant cell contamination in ovarian tissue from patients with breast cancer. Fertility and Sterility. 2011;**95**(6):2158-2161. DOI: 10.1016/j.fertnstert.2010.12.019. Epub 2011 Jan 12

[54] Meirow D, Hardan I, Dor J, Fridman E, Elizur S, Ra'anani H, et al. Searching for evidence of disease and malignant cell contamination in ovarian tissue stored from hematologic cancer patients. Human Reproduction. 2008;**23**(5):1007-1013. DOI: 10.1093/humrep/den055. Epub 2008 Mar 15

[55] Picut CA, Swanson CL, Scully KL, Roseman VC, Parker RF, Remick AK. Ovarian follicle counts using proliferating cell nuclear antigen (PCNA) and semi-automated image analysis in rats. Toxicol Pathololgy. 2008;**36**(5):674-679. DOI: 10.1177/0192623308317428. Epub 2008 May 8

[56] Massin N, Méduri G, Bachelot A, Misrahi M, Kuttenn F, Touraine P. Evaluation of different markers of the ovarian reserve in patients presenting with premature ovarian failure. Molecular and Cellular Endocrinology. 2008;**282**(1-2):95-100. DOI: 10.1016/j.mce.2007.11.017. Epub 2007 Nov 22

[57] Peters IT, Stegehuis PL, Peek R, Boer FL, van Zwet EW, Eggermont J, et al. Noninvasive detection of metastases and follicle density in ovarian tissue using full-field optical coherence tomography. Clincal Cancer Research. 2016;**22**(22):5506-5513. DOI: 10.1158/1078-0432.CCR-16-0288. Epub 2016 May 16

[58] Hu B, Wang R, Wu D, Long R, Ruan J, Jin L, et al. Prospects for fertility

preservation: The ovarian organ function reconstruction techniques for oogenesis, growth and maturation *in vitro*. Frontiers in Physiology. 2023;**14**:1177443. DOI: 10.3389/fphys.2023.1177443

[59] Malo C, Oliván S, Ochoa I, Shikanov A. In vitro growth of human follicles: Current and future perspectives. International Journal of Molecular Sciences. 2024;**25**(3):1510. DOI: 10.3390/ijms25031510

[60] Canosa S, Revelli A, Gennarelli G, Cormio G, Loizzi V, Arezzo F, et al. Innovative strategies for fertility preservation in female cancer survivors: New hope from artificial ovary construction and stem cell-derived neo-folliculogenesis. Healthcare (Basel). 2023;**11**(20):2748. DOI: 10.3390/healthcare11202748

Chapter 4

Expanding the Role of BNIP3 in Autophagy: Hypoxia-Induced Primordial Follicle Loss and Perspectives for Ischemia-Reperfusion Injury in Ovarian Tissue Transplantation

Feng-xia Liu, Zhong Lin and Ka-li Huang

Abstract

Ovarian tissue transplantation (OTT) has become an increasingly important fertility preservation strategy for young women facing gonadotoxic treatments, particularly cancer therapies. Despite its capacity to restore both fertility and endocrine function, OTT outcomes are hindered by the substantial loss of primordial follicles due to ischemic injury after transplantation. This manuscript explores the underlying molecular mechanisms driving follicle depletion, with a specific focus on the role of BNIP3-mediated autophagy and mitophagy. Primordial follicles, established prenatally, are acutely vulnerable to metabolic stress, hypoxia, and subsequent ischemia-reperfusion events that disrupt mitochondrial function and cellular homeostasis in ovarian grafts. BNIP3, a hypoxia-responsive protein, emerges as a central regulator linking hypoxic stress to mitochondrial dynamics, autophagic pathways, and granulosa cell fate in the post-transplant microenvironment. Experimental evidence from in vivo and cellular models highlights the dual role of BNIP3-driven autophagy: initially promoting cell survival under moderate stress, but contributing to excessive follicle loss when overactivated. Pharmacological inhibition of autophagy reveals potential for mitigating follicle attrition, yet important mechanistic questions remain regarding the switch from cell survival to cell death pathways. Understanding the spatiotemporal dynamics and signaling cascades of BNIP3, autophagy, and mitophagy under ischemic conditions may open new avenues for targeted interventions, ultimately improving ovarian reserve preservation and clinical outcomes following OTT.

Keywords: ovarian tissue transplantation, fertility preservation, primordial follicle loss, BNIP3, autophagy, mitophagy, ischemia injury, granulosa cells

1. Introduction

Fertility preservation (FP) is becoming an increasingly important consideration for women whose reproductive capacity has been prematurely compromised due to disease or gonadotoxic therapies. It offers these women renewed opportunities to conceive, carrying significant societal implications. In recent years, the burden of cancer in young women has grown markedly [1, 2]. According to global cancer statistics, the overall incidence rate of cancer among women reached 186.2 per 100,000 in 2022, with approximately 9.658 million new cases reported [3]. In 2020 alone, nearly 900,000 women aged 0–39 were newly diagnosed with cancer worldwide [4]. These epidemiological trends and rising cancer survival rates among young females underscore the growing demand for FP strategies.

Ovarian tissue transplantation (OTT) has emerged as a distinctive FP strategy. From 2018 to 2020, the American Society of Clinical Oncology and the European Society of Human Reproduction and Embryology issued clinical guidelines endorsing OTT as an effective FP method suitable for clinical use [5, 6]. The OTT procedure involves the surgical retrieval of ovarian tissue, preparation of ovarian cortical strips for cryopreservation, and subsequent transplantation of the tissue after appropriate thawing. Compared with other FP techniques, OTT offers several unique advantages [7]: (1) it preserves both fertility and ovarian endocrine function; (2) it eliminates the need for ovarian stimulation prior to transplantation, thus making it suitable for prepubertal girls and women who require urgent cancer treatment; (3) it enables the transplantation of a large quantity of primordial follicles in a single procedure; and (4) it permits repeated transplantations, which can further increase the cumulative pregnancy rate. OTT has demonstrated substantial effectiveness, with more than 200 reported live births globally—pregnancy rates exceeding 41% and live birth rates ranging from 21.6% to 30% [8]. Moreover, restoration of endocrine function has been achieved in nearly all transplanted patients [9].

Despite these positive developments, several limitations persist. The most prominent concern is the significant loss of primordial follicles observed shortly after transplantation. Alongside this predominant challenge, OTT technology faces other important obstacles in practical applications [7, 10, 11]. For instance, the process of ovarian tissue cryopreservation necessitates precise regulation of freezing and thawing rates to prevent ice crystal-induced cellular damage. In cancer survivors, there is the added concern that transplanted ovarian tissue may contain residual microscopic tumors or premalignant cells, posing a potential risk of disease recurrence—a critical safety issue in current OTT practice. Additionally, the translation of foundational research into clinical protocols remains challenging. Although OTT has benefited tremendously from animal models, interspecies physiological differences—such as in hormonal environments, signaling pathways, and growth factor profiles—may limit the direct applicability of preclinical results to humans.

Primordial follicles, established prenatally, constitute the foundation of the ovarian reserve and are subject to continuous, irreversible depletion throughout a woman's life. The unpredictability and severity of this initial follicular loss compromise the long-term efficacy of OTT. Several procedural steps—including tissue excision, processing, cryopreservation, thawing, and autologous transplantation—can contribute to follicular loss. Nonetheless, it is estimated that 75–80% of primordial follicle depletion occurs predominantly during the early period following OTT. Gavish et al. reported that ovarian grafts harvested on day 3 post-transplantation—across multiple species including marmosets, cattle, and humans—suffered an 83–92% loss of primordial follicles, with little further decline thereafter [12]. Unlike transplantation of other organs, OTT does not require vascular anastomosis. Instead, post-transplant blood perfusion depends on the formation of new vascular networks. Consequently, before revascularization is established, ovarian tissue endures extensive and severe ischemic injury. Current understanding suggests that ischemia following OTT activates various downstream mechanisms leading to excessive primordial follicle loss [13]. However, the precise pathways by which ischemic events translate into follicular depletion remain incompletely understood. Notably, attempts to ameliorate follicle loss by simply shortening the ischemic duration or improving the ischemic microenvironment—such as through the enhancement of angiogenic factors or application of bioengineering strategies—have thus far proven insufficient [14–17]. These findings indicate that strategies focused solely on vascular and microenvironmental factors do not fully resolve the issue of follicle loss; instead, it is likely that ischemic stress triggers metabolic dysregulation and the activation of cell death pathways, centrally contributing to the depletion of the primordial follicle pool.

2. Mechanisms of primordial follicle loss after OTT

Compared to the transplantation of other solid organs such as the liver, kidney, or heart, OTT uniquely does not typically require vascular anastomosis, owing to the distinct physiological characteristics of ovarian tissue. The ovary, as an organ inherently adapted to hypoxic conditions, can withstand a certain degree of reduced oxygen supply; indeed, moderate hypoxia may even facilitate follicular growth and development [18]. As a result, transplanted ovarian tissue is capable of surviving for a limited period without immediate vascular reconnection, with its initial blood supply relying primarily on diffusion from the surrounding host tissue until neovascularization is established [13].

In the early phase following transplantation, before the formation of new blood vessels, the ovarian graft exists in an avascular state and depends on the diffusion of oxygen and nutrients from adjacent tissues. During this period, the graft experiences pronounced ischemia and hypoxia. As vascularization progresses, the tissue transitions into an ischemia-reperfusion phase, wherein restoration of blood flow and oxygen supply paradoxically leads to the generation of large amounts of reactive oxygen species (ROS) and heightened inflammatory responses. These pathophysiological changes trigger oxidative stress, tissue injury, and activate multiple cell death pathways within the graft [14]. Granulosa cells play a pivotal role in this context. As the somatic cells enveloping the oocyte, granulosa cells maintain intercellular communication through gap junctions, regulate the oocyte's energy metabolism and development, and influence critical processes such as follicular atresia [19]. Owing to their higher metabolic activity compared to oocytes, granulosa cells are extremely sensitive to alterations in the graft microenvironment. Consequently, they are rapidly affected by ischemic insults, rendering them particularly susceptible during the early hypoxic and subsequent reperfusion stages. This hypersensitivity likely contributes significantly to the massive depletion of primordial follicles seen after OTT, as the compromised granulosa cell environment can no longer support follicular survival.

Ischemic injury during OTT occurs primarily in two critical periods: the initial ischemic-hypoxic phase and the subsequent ischemia-reperfusion phase [20]. Dynamic monitoring studies have shown that in both human and mouse ovarian grafts, organized vascular networks begin to form around the primordial follicles and the ovarian periphery between 3 and 5 days post-transplantation, marking the shift from profound hypoxia to the onset of reperfusion [21, 22]. The timeline of revascularization varies by species, occurring as early as day 3 in mice, by day 7 in rats, and generally requiring about 5 days in humans [23].

As previously discussed, this interval also corresponds to the period of greatest primordial follicle loss. Integrating histopathological observations and mechanistic insights, it can be concluded that ischemic-hypoxic injury and the ensuing reperfusion damage constitute the key factors driving the extensive loss of primordial follicles during OTT.

3. Metabolic stress, mitochondrial dynamics, and autophagy in OTT

Within ovarian grafts following OTT, hypoxia and reperfusion coexist, fashioning a complex microenvironment fraught with metabolic challenge. Following ischemic-hypoxic insult, mitochondrial dysfunction results in a significant reduction in ATP production, triggering a metabolic switch to anaerobic glycolysis. This switch leads to lactate accumulation and a decline in intracellular pH, creating an acidic environment that promotes the buildup of potentially harmful metabolic intermediates like succinate [24]. In response, cells activate adaptive mechanisms, such as increased mitochondrial fusion and fission or induced autophagy to clear damaged organelles. During the subsequent ischemia-reperfusion phase, restoration of oxygen and blood flow induces the rapid oxidation of previously accumulated succinate, generating abundant ROS that damage DNA, proteins, and membrane lipids, ultimately leading to mitochondrial dysfunction characterized by compromised membrane potential, impaired fusion and fission, and defective mitophagy [25]. Mitochondria thus serve as both arbiters of energy and principal sources of ROS, occupying a pivotal role in shaping cell fate under ischemic and reperfusion stress.

The canonical autophagy pathway includes four key steps: autophagosome formation and elongation, lysosome fusion, substrate recognition, and cargo degradation, all orchestrated by autophagy-related genes (ATGs) [26, 27]. Beyond the ATG machinery, autophagy is also modulated by several key signaling pathways, notably the AMPK/mTOR and PI3K/AKT axes, which sense and respond to cellular energy status and various stressors. In hypoxic conditions, hypoxia-inducible factor 1α (HIF-1α) emerges as a central regulator, orchestrating the transcription of ATGs and activating mitophagy mediators such as BNIP3 and NIX, thus facilitating the selective clearance of dysfunctional mitochondria [28]. Mitophagy, a selective autophagy subtype, removes damaged mitochondria to maintain energy balance and cell survival. Through mitochondrial fusion and fission, mitophagy ensures quality control [29]. Under ischemia-hypoxia or ischemia-reperfusion, mitochondria become vulnerable, triggering membrane depolarization and mitophagy pathways, initiated via two main routes [30, 31]: (1) The ubiquitin-dependent pathway: PINK1 accumulation on damaged mitochondria activates Parkin, which ubiquitinates mitochondrial surface proteins. These proteins interact with LC3 and autophagy receptors like p62, promoting mitophagosome formation. (2) The ubiquitin-independent pathway: Receptors such as BNIP3, NIX, and FUNDC1 directly bind LC3 and recruit p62 to form mitophagosomes. These pathways enable autophagy receptors to encapsulate damaged mitochondria into mitophagosomes for lysosomal degradation, preserving mitochondrial integrity and cellular health [32].

In these contexts, autophagy—including mitophagy—acts as a double-edged sword. Moderate hypoxia-induced autophagy may assist cell adaptation by facilitating angiogenesis and clearing injured organelles, thereby reducing follicular loss after transplantation. Conversely, prolonged or severe hypoxia disrupts mitochondrial membrane potential and triggers endoplasmic reticulum stress, instigating a cascade of cell death signals, including autophagic cell death, apoptosis, necrosis, pyroptosis, and others [24, 25, 33–36].

Autophagy plays a key role in follicular development and atresia [37–39]. Genetic mutations in ATGs, such as ATG7, ATG9, and BECN1, reduce the primordial follicle pool and ovarian reserve [40, 41]. For instance, autophagy stimulation in neonatal mice increases primordial follicle numbers, while excessive autophagy, such as due to LSD1 loss, leads to oocyte death. Granulosa cells are particularly sensitive to excessive autophagy, which is strongly linked to follicular atresia [42–44]. Indeed, hypoxia-induced autophagy has been implicated in the elimination of germ cells from mammalian ovaries, and excessive autophagy—especially mitophagy—is strongly associated with follicular atresia [45, 46]. BNIP3, a member of the BCL-2 family, is a critical modulator in this context, promoting mitophagy under hypoxia by dissociating BCL-2 from Beclin 1, initiating autophagosome formation and the selective degradation of dysfunctional mitochondria [47]. While this process reduces ROS accumulation, its excessive activation can exhaust mitochondrial reserves, ultimately leading to ovarian cell death.

Notably, abnormal autophagy or mitophagy dynamics have been documented during ischemia-reperfusion following transplantation in various organs, including the liver, kidney, and lung [29, 48–50]. Recent findings link autophagy dynamics to follicular fate during OTT. Increased autophagic flux is observed in granulosa cells of growing follicles shortly after OTT [51]. Our research also showed rising autophagy in primordial follicle granulosa cells during the first 3 days post-transplant, with autophagy inhibition by 3-methyladenine (3-MA) reducing follicle loss. In a hypoxia model with human granulosa cells, short-term autophagy supported survival, but prolonged autophagy led to dysfunction and death, highlighting the role of BNIP3-mediated mitophagy in granulosa cell survival [52].

Collectively, these observations suggest that autophagy and mitophagy play a dual significant role in ischemia-related excessive primordial follicle loss following OTT, depending on the degree of mitochondrial damage, stress duration, and the balance between mitophagy and mitochondrial biogenesis. Understanding these molecular dynamics offers new perspectives and potential foundations for targeted interventions to better preserve primordial follicles after transplantation.

4. BNIP3: Structure, regulation, and functional role

BNIP3 (Bcl-2/adenovirus E1B 19 kDa interacting protein 3) is a 194-amino acid protein that belongs to the BH3-only subfamily of the Bcl-2 family. It is characterized by its multifunctional capabilities and can exist as either monomers or homodimers, with its function being highly context-dependent [53]. The N-terminal LIR facilitates direct interaction with LC3, playing a critical role in initiating autophagy and mitophagy by promoting the clearance of damaged mitochondria and cellular organelles [54]. Additionally, the PEST sequences serve as degradation signals, modulating BNIP3's stability and activity through proteasomal degradation [55].

Under hypoxic conditions, BNIP3 expression is significantly upregulated, primarily due to the binding of HIF1A to hypoxia-responsive elements (HREs) in its promoter [56, 57]. The atypical BH3 domain enables BNIP3 to interact with Beclin-1 and Bcl-2, thereby regulating both autophagy and apoptosis [58]. The C-terminal transmembrane domain is crucial for mediating cell death, determining subcellular localization, and facilitating homodimerization [47]. When localized to the outer mitochondrial membrane, BNIP3 retains its pro-apoptotic capabilities even in the absence of dimerization [59]. The TM domain anchors BNIP3 to the outer mitochondrial membrane, regulating mitochondrial dynamics and permeability, which leads to cytochrome c release and mitochondrial dysfunction. This anchoring enables BNIP3 to shift to actively triggering mitophagy through its LIR domain, facilitating the selective clearance of damaged mitochondria for quality control and cellular homeostasis [32, 60–62]. Overall, BNIP3 plays a complex and versatile role in apoptosis, autophagy, and mitophagy, with its regulatory functions being significantly influenced by the cellular environment and various stress signals (shown in **Figure 1**).

BNIP3 is essential for cellular health and stress adaptation, notably also linking it to both folliculogenesis and follicular atresia. Owing to the inherently avascular nature of ovarian cortical follicles, granulosa cell proliferation and follicular development occur under relatively hypoxic conditions. During follicular development, the expression of HIF1A and BNIP3, as well as autophagy activity, is significantly upregulated in granulosa cells. This upregulation serves a protective role, safeguarding granulosa cells from apoptosis during the follicular growth phase [18]. Moreover, HIF1A-BNIP3-mediated autophagy plays an essential part in both luteinization and luteolysis of granulosa cells: it protects granulosa-lutein cells from apoptosis in hypoxic environments, while also facilitating cell death during the luteolysis phase [63, 64]. Increasing evidence suggests that BNIP3-driven autophagic death of granulosa cells contribute to follicular atresia and may underlie primordial follicle loss, particularly in instances such as cyclophosphamide-induced ovarian damage [65].

What, then, is the specific role of BNIP3 in follicular survival during OTT?

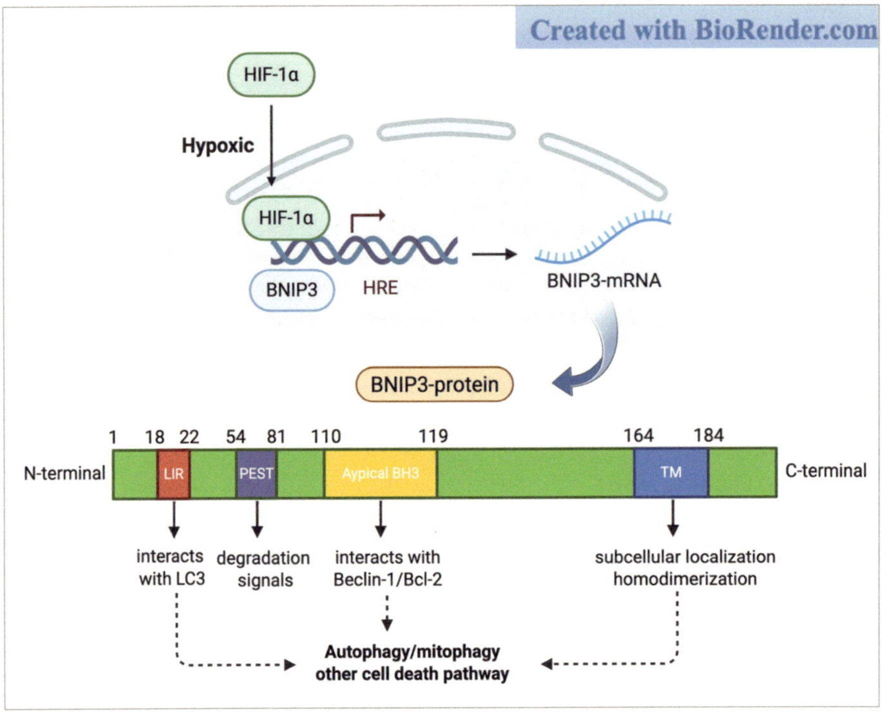

Figure 1.
BNIP3 structure and functions.

5. Experimental evidence of BNIP3-induced follicle loss following OTT

BNIP3-mediated mitophagy is well established as a key mechanism in the cellular response to ischemia-reperfusion injury across multiple tissue types [66–69]. Given the similar ischemia-reperfusion challenges faced in OTT, BNIP3 emerges as a critical regulator in this context as well. Importantly, mere accumulation of BNIP3 in response to hypoxia is not sufficient to induce cell death. Instead, it is prolonged ischemia-reperfusion injury that robustly activates BNIP3, which through downstream signaling cascades—particularly those affecting cellular energy homeostasis—ultimately precipitates cell death. Under conditions of mild hypoxia, mitophagy orchestrated by BNIP3 serves a protective function, maintaining intracellular oxygen homeostasis by eliminating dysfunctional mitochondria and suppressing excessive aerobic respiration. However, when hypoxia surpasses cellular tolerance thresholds, BNIP3-induced mitophagy becomes excessively activated, manifesting as increased fusion of mitophagosomes and lysosomes, amplified autophagic flux, and ultimately the onset of autophagic cell death [62].

Building on this knowledge, emerging studies have begun to clarify the involvement of BNIP3 in primordial follicle loss following OTT. The ischemic microenvironment characteristic of the early post-transplantation period elevates the relevance of BNIP3, given its established regulatory functions in hypoxia- and ischemia/reperfusion-triggered autophagy, mitophagy, and cell death. The interaction between BNIP3 and hypoxia/reperfusion-responsive elements may determine follicular cell survival—shaping whether autophagic or apoptotic pathways predominate, and thus influencing the fate of the ovarian follicle pool. Elucidating the precise role of BNIP3 in this setting not only advances our mechanistic understanding under ischemic stress, but also offers promising new molecular targets for therapeutic intervention to mitigate primordial follicle loss and enhance OTT outcomes.

An in vivo investigation by our team using murine models of ovarian auto-transplantation further substantiates the pivotal role of BNIP3-mediated autophagy in early follicular loss following transplantation. Administration of the autophagy inhibitor 3-MA led to a partial restoration of primordial follicle numbers within the ovarian grafts, while granulosa cells exhibited upregulated BNIP3 expression and increased activation of the autophagy pathway. Subsequent cell experiments confirmed that under hypoxic conditions, BNIP3 activates autophagy through the mTOR/ULK1 pathway. These results provide strong support for the involvement of the hypoxia-BNIP3-mTOR/ULK1 signaling axis in primordial follicle loss after OTT [52]. On the basis of these findings, a potential mechanism was proposed for primordial follicle loss following OTT: After transplantation, both BNIP3 and autophagy are markedly upregulated in granulosa cells of primordial follicles, and this heightened activity correlates with significant follicle loss. Notably, pharmacological inhibition of autophagy effectively mitigates primordial follicle depletion, underscoring the pivotal regulatory role of BNIP3—functioning within the HIF1A-BNIP3-mTOR/ULK1 axis—in hypoxia-induced cellular autophagy.

6. Unresolved questions and translational directions

These insights shed new light on the molecular events driving primordial follicle loss after OTT and highlight the central role of BNIP3-mediated autophagy as a response to hypoxic stress. Nevertheless, a mechanistic gap persists between BNIP3-induced autophagy and the final trigger for primordial follicle death. It is now well established that BNIP3 is intimately linked to mitochondrial metabolism and regulates diverse cell fate pathways, including autophagy, mitophagy, and cell death processes—including apoptosis, necrosis, and ferroptosis. Whether early ischemia-reperfusion after OTT promotes excessive loss of primordial follicles via BNIP3-driven mitophagy, and how such protective mechanisms ultimately convert to pro-death pathways, are critical scientific questions that warrant in-depth exploration. Dissecting the molecular interplay between BNIP3-induced mitophagy and these death modalities in the OTT setting will be crucial for identifying context-specific intervention points.

To further investigate the role of BNIP3 in the loss of primordial follicles following OTT, CRISPR/Cas9 gene editing technology can be utilized to create a conditional knockout mouse model for BNIP3. Ovarian grafts will be monitored at different time points post-transplantation (e.g., 6, 12, 24, 48, and 72 hours) and compared with those from wild-type mice. The indicators to be assessed include: (1) oxygen partial pressure, the number of new blood vessels, and ROS levels to determine the stage of ischemia or reperfusion in the grafts; (2) the loss of primordial follicles; (3) the expression levels of BNIP3 gene and protein; and (4) the activity of autophagy and mitophagy, as well as changes in ferroptosis and apoptosis. Comparing levels of biomarkers at different time points post-OTT between the BNIP3 knockout group and wild-type mice, and correlating the changes in BNIP3 expression, autophagy/mitophagy, ferroptosis, and apoptosis activity with the loss of primordial follicles would reveal the impact of BNIP3 deficiency on cell survival mechanisms. Beyond traditional experimental techniques, single-cell RNA sequencing could be utilized to analyze mRNA expression profiles of BNIP3 knockout mice and wild-type controls, identifying differentially expressed genes and regulatory pathways related to autophagy, mitophagy, ferroptosis, and apoptosis. Concurrently, metabolomics analysis might provide a comprehensive assessment of the relationship between metabolic changes and cell survival, elucidating the connections between BNIP3, cellular energy metabolism, and oxidative stress, thereby enriching the understanding of the mechanisms underlying BNIP3's role in ischemic injury following ovarian transplantation.

From a translational perspective, targeting BNIP3 as a means to prevent follicle loss holds theoretical appeal. However, several technical challenges persist: (1) the lack of highly specific BNIP3 modulators that do not perturb physiological mitophagy and cellular homeostasis, (2) challenges in targeted drug delivery to ovarian grafts in situ, and (3) the risk of off-target effects, given BNIP3's role in multiple tissues and stress responses. Nevertheless, the application of nanotechnology for targeted delivery holds promise in addressing these challenges.

Emerging nanoregulator technology in OTT has progressed from theoretical conception to a stage supported by experimental evidence. Through multiple animal models (such as sheep and mice), nanotechnology has demonstrated significant effects in inhibiting ice crystal formation, promoting angiogenesis, reducing oxidative stress, and selectively eliminating tumor cells [70]. Researchers have utilized nanotechnology to deliver angiogenic substances (such as nitric oxide, NO), promoting blood vessel formation in transplanted ovarian tissue, or employed nanoregulators with antioxidant properties to clear ROS in tissues, thereby reducing oxidative damage and improving transplantation success rates [71, 72]. Zhang et al. developed AMH-targeted nanobubbles for ultrasound molecular imaging, successfully achieving real-time monitoring of the survival status of transplanted ovarian tissue [73]. Although nanotechnology has not yet been widely applied in clinical settings, experimental results indicate its vast potential and promising prospects in the field of OTT.

The mouse OTT model remains the most widely used preclinical model for OTT [74]. Its advantages are reflected in several aspects: First, mice share a high degree of genomic homology with humans, reaching 99%, and their anatomical structure and physiological functions are highly similar to those of human ovaries, allowing for a good simulation of the physiological and pathological processes of human OTT. Second, the mouse model allows comprehensive assessment of the transplanted ovarian tissue post-transplantation, including histological analysis, angiogenesis density, granulosa cell proliferation activity, and monitoring of hormone levels and estrous cycles, providing multidimensional evidence for evaluating transplantation efficacy. Additionally, the mouse model supports diverse transplantation methods, such as heterotopic transplantation, syngeneic transplantation, and autologous transplantation, offering flexibility in studying different transplantation strategies. It also enables the investigation of specific genes' mechanisms of action during the OTT process or the effects of various intervention drugs on transplantation outcomes through genetic engineering techniques. However, there are certain limitations to the mouse model. Firstly, despite the high genomic homology between mice and humans, there are differences in their physiological environments, which may affect the predictability of transplantation outcomes. For instance, the choice of transplantation site (such as subcutaneous tissue or renal capsule) may yield different effects in mice compared to humans, and the blood supply and microenvironment characteristics of different transplantation sites significantly influence the transplantation results. Secondly, existing assessment standards have not yet been fully standardized, leading to variations in the timing and methods of evaluating transplantation outcomes across different studies, which limits the comparability of research results. Notably, animal experiments face significant challenges in precision translational medicine, as conclusions drawn from animal models do not necessarily apply directly to humans. This limitation highlights the necessity for effective translational strategies to bridge the gap between preclinical findings and clinical applications, ensuring that therapeutic approaches identified through animal research are relevant and safe for human populations.

Looking ahead, integrating multi-omic technologies (such as single-cell transcriptomics, proteomics, and metabolomics) combined with advanced nanotechnology and preclinical models will be instrumental in unraveling complex BNIP3-regulated networks and defining patient-specific risk factors. Furthermore, these platforms can accelerate the screening and validation of novel BNIP3-targeted interventions. Close collaboration between basic researchers and clinicians will be essential to translate these mechanistic insights into clinical strategies, moving from bench to bedside to optimize fertility outcomes in OTT patients.

7. Conclusions

In summary, primordial follicle loss remains the principal challenge limiting the long-term efficacy of OTT for FP in young women undergoing gonadotoxic treatments. Accumulating evidence presented in this chapter highlights that ischemic-hypoxic injury and subsequent ischemia-reperfusion events induce severe metabolic and mitochondrial dysfunction, activating multiple regulated cell death pathways in ovarian grafts. Central to these processes is BNIP3—a hypoxia-responsive adaptor protein—that orchestrates mitophagy and autophagy in granulosa cells under ischemic stress. Experimental data consistently demonstrate that BNIP3-mediated autophagy is markedly upregulated post-OTT and is closely associated with primordial follicle depletion, while pharmacological inhibition of autophagy partially mitigates follicle loss. However, significant mechanistic questions persist regarding the dynamic switch of BNIP3 from a protective to a pro-death role, its interplay with other cell death pathways, and the feasibility of targeting BNIP3 for clinical intervention. Moving forward, detailed investigations leveraging multi-omics approaches and advanced in vitro models are warranted to further unravel the temporal and molecular regulation of BNIP3 in this context. Ultimately, targeting BNIP3-regulated mitophagy holds substantial promise for optimizing OTT outcomes and preserving reproductive potential in affected patients.

Acknowledgements

The authors would like to thank all the members of the research team for their technical assistance and valuable discussions throughout the course of this study.

This work was funded by the self-raised scientific research fund of the Guangxi Zhuang Autonomous Region Health Commission (Grant No. Z-A20240398); the Nanning Qingxiu district self-financed science and technology project—key research and development program (Grant No. 2023ZC001); Guangxi science and technology base and talent project (Grant no. AC22080002); Guangxi key research and development plan project (Grant no. AB22035080).

Conflict of interest

The authors declare no conflict of interest.

Author details

Feng-xia Liu*, Zhong Lin and Ka-li Huang
Department of Reproductive Medicine, Reproductive Hospital of Guangxi Zhuang Autonomous Region, Nanning, Guangxi, P.R. China

*Address all correspondence to: liufengxia34@163.com

References

[1] Jiang X, Tang H, Chen T. Epidemiology of gynecologic cancers in China. Journal of Gynecologic Oncology. 2018;**29**(1):e7. DOI: 10.3802/jgo.2018.29.e7

[2] Zhang SZ, Zhang L, Xie L. Cancer burden in China during 1990-2019: Analysis of the global burden of disease. BioMed Research International. 2022;**2022**:3918045. DOI: 10.1155/2022/3918045

[3] Bray F, Laversanne M, Sung H, et al. Global cancer statistics 2022: GLOBOCAN estimates of incidence and mortality worldwide for 36 cancers in 185 countries. CA: A Cancer Journal for Clinicians. 2024;**74**(3):229-263. DOI: 10.3322/caac.21834

[4] International Agency for Research on Cancer WHO. Estimated Number of New Cases in 2020, All Cancers, Females, Ages 0-39 [Z]. 2020. Available from: https://gco.iarc.fr/today/home

[5] Oktay K, Harvey BE, Partridge AH, et al. Fertility preservation in patients with cancer: ASCO clinical practice guideline update. Journal of Clinical Oncology. 2018;**36**(19):1994-2001. DOI: 10.1200/jco.2018.78.1914

[6] Anderson RA, Amant F, Braat D, et al. ESHRE guideline: Female fertility preservation. Human Reproduction Open. 2020;**2020**(4):hoaa052. DOI: 10.1093/hropen/hoaa052

[7] Thuwanut P, Leonel ECR, Rocha Ruiz TF, et al. Human ovarian tissue xenotransplantation: Advancements, challenges, and future perspectives. Human Reproduction. 2025;**40**(3):410-419. DOI: 10.1093/humrep/deae291

[8] Kristensen SG, Olesen H, Zeuthen MC, et al. Revascularization of human ovarian grafts is equally efficient from both sides of the cortex tissue. Reproductive Biomedicine Online. 2022;**44**(6):991-994. DOI: 10.1016/j.rbmo.2022.02.009

[9] Diaz-Garcia C, Domingo J, Garcia-Velasco JA, et al. Oocyte vitrification versus ovarian cortex transplantation in fertility preservation for adult women undergoing gonadotoxic treatments: A prospective cohort study. Fertility and Sterility. 2018;**109**(3):478-85.e2. DOI: 10.1016/j.fertnstert.2017.11.018

[10] Dunlop CE, Anderson RA. Clinical dilemmas in ovarian tissue cryopreservation. Fertility and Sterility. 2024;**122**(4):559-564. DOI: 10.1016/j.fertnstert.2024.05.167

[11] Anderson RA, Baird DT. The development of ovarian tissue cryopreservation in Edinburgh: Translation from a rodent model through validation in a large mammal and then into clinical practice. Acta Obstetricia et Gynecologica Scandinavica. 2019;**98**(5):545-549. DOI: 10.1111/aogs.13560

[12] Gavish Z, Spector I, Peer G, et al. Follicle activation is a significant and immediate cause of follicle loss after ovarian tissue transplantation. Journal of Assisted Reproduction and Genetics. 2018;**35**(1):61-69. DOI: 10.1007/s10815-017-1079-z

[13] Roness H, Meirow D. Fertility preservation: Follicle reserve loss in ovarian tissue transplantation. Reproduction. 2019;**158**(5):F35-f44. DOI: 10.1530/rep-19-0097

[14] Cacciottola L, Donnez J, Dolmans MM. Ovarian tissue damage

after grafting: Systematic review of strategies to improve follicle outcomes. Reproductive Biomedicine Online. 2021;**43**(3):351-369. DOI: 10.1016/j.rbmo.2021.06.019

[15] Mehdinia Z, Ashrafi M, Fathi R, et al. Restoration of estrous cycles by co-transplantation of mouse ovarian tissue with MSCs. Cell and Tissue Research. 2020;**381**(3):509-525. DOI: 10.1007/s00441-020-03204-x

[16] Olesen H, Pors SE, Adrados CS, et al. Effects of needle puncturing on re-vascularization and follicle survival in xenotransplanted human ovarian tissue. Reproductive Biology and Endocrinology. 2023;**21**(1):28. DOI: 10.1186/s12958-023-01081-x

[17] Manavella DD, Cacciottola L, Payen VL, et al. Adipose tissue-derived stem cells boost vascularization in grafted ovarian tissue by growth factor secretion and differentiation into endothelial cell lineages. Molecular Human Reproduction. 2019;**25**(4):184-193. DOI: 10.1093/molehr/gaz008

[18] Tang Z, Xu R, Zhang Z, et al. HIF-1α protects granulosa cells from hypoxia-induced apoptosis during follicular development by inducing autophagy. Frontiers in Cell and Development Biology. 2021;**9**:631016. DOI: 10.3389/fcell.2021.631016

[19] Liu X, Mai H, Chen P, et al. Comparative analyses in transcriptome of human granulosa cells and follicular fluid micro-environment between poor ovarian responders with conventional controlled ovarian or mild ovarian stimulations. Reproductive Biology and Endocrinology. 2022;**20**(1):54. DOI: 10.1186/s12958-022-00926-1

[20] Mamsen LS, Olesen H, Pors SE, et al. Effects of Er:YAG laser treatment on re-vascularization and follicle survival in frozen/thawed human ovarian cortex transplanted to immunodeficient mice. Journal of Assisted Reproduction and Genetics. 2021;**38**(10):2745-2756. DOI: 10.1007/s10815-021-02292-0

[21] Van Eyck AS, Jordan BF, Gallez B, et al. Electron paramagnetic resonance as a tool to evaluate human ovarian tissue reoxygenation after xenografting. Fertility and Sterility. 2009;**92**(1):374-381. DOI: 10.1016/j.fertnstert.2008.05.012

[22] Cheng J, Ruan X, Li Y, et al. Effects of hypoxia-preconditioned HucMSCs on neovascularization and follicle survival in frozen/thawed human ovarian cortex transplanted to immunodeficient mice. Stem Cell Research & Therapy. 2022;**13**(1):474. DOI: 10.1186/s13287-022-03167-6

[23] Grosbois J, Devos M, Demeestere I. Implications of nonphysiological ovarian primordial follicle activation for fertility preservation. Endocrine Reviews. 2020;**41**(6):bnaa020. DOI: 10.1210/endrev/bnaa020

[24] Dugbartey GJ. Cellular and molecular mechanisms of cell damage and cell death in ischemia-reperfusion injury in organ transplantation. Molecular Biology Reports. 2024;**51**(1):473. DOI: 10.1007/s11033-024-09261-7

[25] Milliken AS, Kulkarni CA, Brookes PS. Acid enhancement of ROS generation by complex-I reverse electron transport is balanced by acid inhibition of complex-II: Relevance for tissue reperfusion injury. Redox Biology. 2020;**37**:101733. DOI: 10.1016/j.redox.2020.101733

[26] Liu S, Yao S, Yang H, et al. Autophagy: Regulator of cell death. Cell Death & Disease. 2023;**14**(10):648. DOI: 10.1038/s41419-023-06154-8

[27] Klionsky DJ, Abdel-Aziz AK, Abdelfatah S, et al. Guidelines for the use and interpretation of assays for monitoring autophagy (4th edition) (1). Autophagy. 2021;**17**(1):1-382. DOI: 10.1080/15548627.2020.1797280

[28] Zhang J, Ney PA. Role of BNIP3 and NIX in cell death, autophagy, and mitophagy. Cell Death and Differentiation. 2009;**16**(7):939-946. DOI: 10.1038/cdd.2009.16

[29] Granata S, Votrico V, Spadaccino F, et al. Oxidative stress and ischemia/reperfusion injury in kidney transplantation: Focus on ferroptosis, mitophagy and new antioxidants. Antioxidants (Basel). 2022;**11**(4):769. DOI: 10.3390/antiox11040769

[30] Vera-Ramirez L. Cell-intrinsic survival signals. The role of autophagy in metastatic dissemination and tumor cell dormancy. Seminars in Cancer Biology. 2020;**60**:28-40. DOI: 10.1016/j.semcancer.2019.07.027

[31] Lu Y, Li Z, Zhang S, et al. Cellular mitophagy: Mechanism, roles in diseases and small molecule pharmacological regulation. Theranostics. 2023;**13**(2):736-766. DOI: 10.7150/thno.79876

[32] Onishi M, Yamano K, Sato M, et al. Molecular mechanisms and physiological functions of mitophagy. The EMBO Journal. 2021;**40**(3):e104705. DOI: 10.15252/embj.2020104705

[33] Eltzschig HK, Eckle T. Ischemia and reperfusion—From mechanism to translation. Nature Medicine. 2011;**17**(11):1391-1401. DOI: 10.1038/nm.2507

[34] Huang R, Zhang C, Xiang Z, et al. Role of mitochondria in renal ischemia-reperfusion injury. The FEBS Journal. 2024;**291**(24):5365-5378. DOI: 10.1111/febs.17130

[35] Przyklenk K, Dong Y, Undyala VV, Whittaker P. Autophagy as a therapeutic target for ischaemia/reperfusion injury? Concepts, controversies, and challenges. Cardiovascular Research. 2012;**94**(2):197-205. DOI: 10.1093/cvr/cvr358

[36] Ying H, Shi L, Zhang S. Research progress on mechanism of follicle injury after ovarian tissue transplantation and protective strategies. Zhejiang Da Xue Xue Bao. Yi Xue Ban. 2024;**53**(3):321-330. DOI: 10.3724/zdxbyxb-2023-0566

[37] Zheng Y, Ma L, Liu N, et al. Autophagy and apoptosis of porcine ovarian granulosa cells during follicular development. Animals (Basel). 2019;**9**(12):1111. DOI: 10.3390/ani9121111

[38] Zhou J, Peng X, Mei S. Autophagy in ovarian follicular development and atresia. International Journal of Biological Sciences. 2019;**15**(4):726-737. DOI: 10.7150/ijbs.30369

[39] Leopardo NP, Velazquez ME, Cortasa S, et al. A dual death/survival role of autophagy in the adult ovary of *Lagostomus maximus* (Mammalia-Rodentia). PLoS ONE. 2020;**15**(5):e0232819. DOI: 10.1371/journal.pone.0232819

[40] Umeno K, Sasaki A, Kimura N. The impact of oocyte death on mouse primordial follicle formation and ovarian reserve. Reproductive Medicine and Biology. 2022;**21**(1):e12489. DOI: 10.1002/rmb2.12489

[41] Delcour C, Amazit L, Patino LC, et al. ATG7 and ATG9A loss-of-function variants trigger autophagy impairment and ovarian failure. Genetics in

Medicine. 2019;**21**(4):930-938. DOI: 10.1038/s41436-018-0287-y

[42] Watanabe R, Kimura N. Non-suckling starvation of neonatal mice promotes primordial follicle formation with activation of ovarian autophagy. The Journal of Reproduction and Development. 2018;**64**(1):89-94. DOI: 10.1262/jrd.2017-126

[43] Watanabe R, Sasaki S, Kimura N. Activation of autophagy in early neonatal mice increases primordial follicle number and improves lifelong fertility†. Biology of Reproduction. 2020;**102**(2):399-411. DOI: 10.1093/biolre/ioz179

[44] Choi JY, Jo MW, Lee EY, et al. The role of autophagy in follicular development and atresia in rat granulosa cells. Fertility and Sterility. 2010;**93**(8):2532-2537. DOI: 10.1016/j.fertnstert.2009.11.021

[45] He M, Zhang T, Zhu Z, et al. LSD1 contributes to programmed oocyte death by regulating the transcription of autophagy adaptor SQSTM1/p62. Aging Cell. 2020;**19**(3):e13102. DOI: 10.1111/acel.13102

[46] Yadav AK, Yadav PK, Chaudhary GR, et al. Autophagy in hypoxic ovary. Cellular and Molecular Life Sciences. 2019;**76**(17):3311-3322. DOI: 10.1007/s00018-019-03122-4

[47] Field JT, Gordon JW. BNIP3 and Nix: Atypical regulators of cell fate. Biochimica et Biophysica Acta, Molecular Cell Research. 2022;**1869**(10):119325. DOI: 10.1016/j.bbamcr.2022.119325

[48] Liu WC, Chen SB, Liu S, et al. Inhibition of mitochondrial autophagy protects donor lungs for lung transplantation against ischaemia-reperfusion injury in rats via the mTOR pathway. Journal of Cellular and Molecular Medicine. 2019;**23**(5):3190-3201. DOI: 10.1111/jcmm.14177

[49] Dar WA, Sullivan E, Bynon JS, et al. Ischaemia reperfusion injury in liver transplantation: Cellular and molecular mechanisms. Liver International. 2019;**39**(5):788-801. DOI: 10.1111/liv.14091

[50] Liu Q, Krishnasamy Y, Rehman H, et al. Disrupted renal mitochondrial homeostasis after liver transplantation in rats. PLoS ONE. 2015;**10**(10):e0140906. DOI: 10.1371/journal.pone.0140906

[51] Xu Z. Autophagy phenomenon in mice ovaries following transplantation. Theriogenology. 2023;**195**:40-45. DOI: 10.1016/j.theriogenology.2022.10.018

[52] Liu F, Li M. BNIP3-mediated autophagy via the mTOR/ULK1 pathway induces primordial follicle loss after ovarian tissue transplantation. Journal of Assisted Reproduction and Genetics. 2023;**40**(3):491-508. DOI: 10.1007/s10815-023-02765-4

[53] Gorbunova AS, Yapryntseva MA, Denisenko TV, Zhivotovsky B. BNIP3 in lung cancer: To kill or rescue? Cancers (Basel). 2020;**12**(11):3390. DOI: 10.3390/cancers12113390

[54] Hanna RA, Quinsay MN, Orogo AM, et al. Microtubule-associated protein 1 light chain 3 (LC3) interacts with Bnip3 protein to selectively remove endoplasmic reticulum and mitochondria via autophagy. The Journal of Biological Chemistry. 2012;**287**(23):19094-19104. DOI: 10.1074/jbc.M111.322933

[55] Rogers S, Wells R, Rechsteiner M. Amino acid sequences common to rapidly degraded proteins: The PEST hypothesis. Science. 1986;**234**(4774):364-368. DOI: 10.1126/science.2876518

[56] Fu ZJ, Wang ZY, Xu L, et al. HIF-1α-BNIP3-mediated mitophagy in tubular cells protects against renal ischemia/reperfusion injury. Redox Biology. 2020;**36**:101671. DOI: 10.1016/j.redox.2020.101671

[57] Yang Y, Lu H, Chen C, et al. HIF-1 interacts with TRIM28 and DNA-PK to release paused RNA polymerase II and activate target gene transcription in response to hypoxia. Nature Communications. 2022;**13**(1):316. DOI: 10.1038/s41467-021-27944-8

[58] Chinnadurai G, Vijayalingam S, Gibson SB. BNIP3 subfamily BH3-only proteins: Mitochondrial stress sensors in normal and pathological functions. Oncogene. 2008;**27**(Suppl. 1):S114-S127. DOI: 10.1038/onc.2009.49

[59] Ray R, Chen G, Vande Velde C, et al. BNIP3 heterodimerizes with Bcl-2/Bcl-X(L) and induces cell death independent of a Bcl-2 homology 3 (BH3) domain at both mitochondrial and nonmitochondrial sites. The Journal of Biological Chemistry. 2000;**275**(2):1439-1448. DOI: 10.1074/jbc.275.2.1439

[60] Chen Y, Yan Q, Xu Y, et al. BNIP3-mediated autophagy induced inflammatory response and inhibited VEGF expression in cultured retinal pigment epithelium cells under hypoxia. Current Molecular Medicine. 2019;**19**(6):395-404. DOI: 10.2174/1566524019666190509105502

[61] Madhu V, Hernandez-Meadows M, Boneski PK, et al. The mitophagy receptor BNIP3 is critical for the regulation of metabolic homeostasis and mitochondrial function in the nucleus pulposus cells of the intervertebral disc. Autophagy. 2023;**19**(6):1821-1843. DOI: 10.1080/15548627.2022.2162245

[62] Niemi NM, Friedman JR. Coordinating BNIP3/NIX-mediated mitophagy in space and time. Biochemical Society Transactions. 2024;**52**(5):1969-1979. DOI: 10.1042/bst20221364

[63] Tang Z, Zhang Z, Lin Q, et al. HIF-1α/BNIP3-mediated autophagy contributes to the luteinization of granulosa cells during the formation of corpus luteum. Frontiers in Cell and Development Biology. 2020;**8**:619924. DOI: 10.3389/fcell.2020.619924

[64] Tang Z, Chen J, Zhang Z, et al. HIF-1α activation promotes luteolysis by enhancing ROS levels in the corpus luteum of pseudopregnant rats. Oxidative Medicine and Cellular Longevity. 2021;**2021**:1764929. DOI: 10.1155/2021/1764929

[65] Zhu F, Gao J, Zeng F, et al. Hyperoside protects against cyclophosphamide induced ovarian damage and reduced fertility by suppressing HIF-1α/BNIP3-mediated autophagy. Biomedicine & Pharmacotherapy. 2022;**156**:113743. DOI: 10.1016/j.biopha.2022.113743

[66] Xie W, Zhu T, Zhang S, Sun X. Protective effects of Gypenoside XVII against cerebral ischemia/reperfusion injury via SIRT1-FOXO3A- and Hif1a-BNIP3-mediated mitochondrial autophagy. Journal of Translational Medicine. 2022;**20**(1):622. DOI: 10.1186/s12967-022-03830-9

[67] Yu Q, Fu W, Fu Y, et al. BNIP3 as a potential biomarker for the identification of prognosis and diagnosis in solid tumours. Molecular Cancer. 2023;**22**(1):143. DOI: 10.1186/s12943-023-01808-9

[68] Marzook H, Gupta A, Jayakumar MN, et al. GSK-3α-BNIP3 axis promotes mitophagy in human

cardiomyocytes under hypoxia. Free Radical Biology & Medicine. 2024;**221**:235-244. DOI: 10.1016/j.freeradbiomed.2024.05.041

[69] Lee TL, Shen WC, Chen YC, et al. Mir221- and Mir222-enriched adsc-exosomes mitigate PM exposure-exacerbated cardiac ischemia-reperfusion injury through the modulation of the BNIP3-MAP1LC3B-BBC3/PUMA pathway. Autophagy. 2025;**21**(2):374-393. DOI: 10.1080/15548627.2024.2395799

[70] Jiang M, Zhang GH, Yu Y, et al. De novo design of a nanoregulator for the dynamic restoration of ovarian tissue in cryopreservation and transplantation. Journal of Nanobiotechnology. 2024;**22**(1):330. DOI: 10.1186/s12951-024-02602-5

[71] Kang Y, Kim J, Park J, et al. Tumor vasodilation by N-heterocyclic carbene-based nitric oxide delivery triggered by high-intensity focused ultrasound and enhanced drug homing to tumor sites for anti-cancer therapy. Biomaterials. 2019;**217**:119297. DOI: 10.1016/j.biomaterials.2019.119297

[72] Lautner G, Meyerhoff ME, Schwendeman SP. Biodegradable poly(lactic-co-glycolic acid) microspheres loaded with S-nitroso-N-acetyl-d-penicillamine for controlled nitric oxide delivery. Journal of Controlled Release. 2016;**225**:133-139. DOI: 10.1016/j.jconrel.2015.12.056

[73] Zhang S, Di N, Tayier B, et al. Early evaluation of survival of the transplanted ovaries through ultrasound molecular imaging via targeted nanobubbles. Biomaterials Science. 2020;**8**:5402-5414. DOI: 10.1039/d0bm01125h

[74] Liu FX, Lin Z, Huang KL. Developing mouse models for ovarian tissue transplantation and xenotransplantation: A review. Medical Science Monitor. 2025;**31**:e946386. DOI: 10.12659/MSM.946386

Chapter 5

Fertility Preservation in Hematological Malignancies: A Growing Imperative

Georgi Stamenov and Kameliya Kostadinova

Abstract

Advances in successful treatment for hematological malignancies have dramatically improved patient survival, making fertility preservation a growing imperative for individuals of reproductive age. This review outlines key aspects of oncofertility, focusing on the mechanisms of treatment-induced damage, critical risk factors, and established strategies for preserving fertility in this patient population. Chemotherapy and radiotherapy, as forms of cytotoxic therapy, are known to induce gonadotoxicity by primarily affecting rapidly dividing ovarian cells, which results in the paradoxical depletion of the primordial follicle reserve. The risk of premature ovarian insufficiency (POI) is multifactorial, with patient age at the time of treatment, the specific chemotherapy regimen (e.g., alkylating agents), and the need for hematopoietic stem cell transplantation (HSCT) being the most critical predictors. Oocyte or embryo cryopreservation following a short protocol controlled ovarian stimulation the gold standard as a fertility preservation method. While medical advances offer viable options, a significant gap in physician-patient communication regarding fertility risks persists. The effective collaboration between hemato-oncologists and reproductive specialists is paramount for successful fertility preservation and enables patients to make informed decisions about their future reproductive health.

Keywords: female fertility, hematology malignancies, gonadotoxicity, premature ovarian insufficiency, fertility preservation

1. Introduction

Advances in the successful treatment of various hematological diseases have dramatically improved patient survival rates, making the crucial question of fertility preservation a paramount concern for individuals of reproductive age. According to data from the National Institutes of Health (NIH), five-year survival rates are now substantial, reaching 70% for chronic myeloid leukemia, 72% for acute lymphoblastic leukemia, and an impressive 88.9% for Hodgkin's lymphoma [1]. The Center for International Blood and Marrow Transplant Research (CIBMTR) has documented a constant rise in allogeneic hematopoietic stem cell transplantation (AlloHSCT), with projections estimating 500,000 AlloHSCT survivors by 2030 [2]. These improved treatment outcomes have led to a significant reduction in mortality rates among young adults.

However, the reproductive system is particularly susceptible to the adverse effects of both cancer itself and its aggressive treatments. The use of cytotoxic treatments, including radiotherapy, may reduce reproductive capacity and potentially lead to permanent infertility in patients [3]. This damage is further complicated by secondary factors such as graft-versus-host disease (GvHD) after AlloHSCT [4] and the presence of post-transfusion iron overload. Female cancer survivors exhibit a considerably reduced rate of childbirth (18% lower) compared to the general population, alongside a 36-fold lower likelihood of achieving conception following AlloHSCT [5, 6].

Several mechanisms contribute to this cytotoxic damage to the reproductive system. The extent of ovarian damage is multifaceted, depending on the specific cancer type, the types and doses of chemotherapy and radiotherapy used, as well as the patient's age and baseline ovarian reserve. A critical distinction lies in the unique ontogenetic development of the female reproductive system: females are born with a finite number of oocytes, peaking at around 7 million by 20 weeks of fetal development. Ovarian follicles naturally undergo continuous atresia; their count decreases to roughly 1 million by birth and continues to diminish until menopause, which is defined by the exhaustion of the oocyte supply [7]. Consequently, unlike the virtually unlimited sperm production in men (provided spermatogonial stem cells are present), the fixed number of oocytes in women presents a greater challenge for medical teams in preserving their reproductive potential compared to men.

Given this critical relationship, the term "oncofertility" has arisen to define a crucial interdisciplinary area that addresses the overlap between oncology and reproductive medicine [8]. It employs a comprehensive multidisciplinary approach that necessitates robust coordination and collaboration among hemato-oncologists, gynecologists, reproductive biologists, and patients. This collaborative model has been shown to significantly increase the likelihood of conception in young cancer patients. The term "oncofertility" was notably coined in 2006 by Professor Teresa Woodruff, the founder and director of the Oncofertility Consortium at Northwestern University, Chicago, Illinois, USA.

In the subsequent sections, we will delve into specific features related to hematological diseases and the various possibilities for preserving fertility.

2. Hematological malignancies and female fertility: An overview

Hematological malignancies account for a notable 7–9% of all new cancer diagnoses and deaths in women. Among women of reproductive age, the most common diagnoses include acute lymphoblastic leukemia, acute myeloid leukemia, non-Hodgkin lymphoma (NHL), and Hodgkin lymphoma. Current knowledge regarding the impact of cytotoxic therapies on the gonads of premenopausal women is predominantly derived from comprehensive studies conducted in lymphoma patients [9]. Our understanding of the impact of cytotoxic therapies on the gonads of premenopausal women is largely based on extensive studies of lymphoma patients.

2.1 Fertility concerns in lymphoma and acute leukemias

While initial, standard treatment regimens for these specific diseases might carry a low inherent risk of gonadotoxicity, it is crucial to consider each patient's unique situation. Factors like the potential for the cancer to resist therapy initially, the chance of relapse, the need for more intensive treatments, or the possibility of a stem cell transplantation can significantly increase the risk to fertility. These considerations necessitate a proactive approach to fertility preservation.

2.2 Fertility in other hematological malignancies

Other forms of blood cancer, like chronic lymphocytic leukemia and multiple myeloma, typically affect older individuals (usually over 50, often after menopause), so fertility concerns are generally not a primary consideration in these cases. The standard treatments for Myeloproliferative Neoplasms do not involve gonadotoxic therapies. Therefore, unless a patient is considering a stem cell transplant, a detailed discussion about fertility preservation is usually not necessary for MPNs.

3. Mechanisms of gonadotoxicity in cancer treatment

The impact of cancer therapies on female fertility is a significant concern, primarily manifesting as POI. While various mechanisms of gonadotoxicity have been proposed for different chemotherapy agents, the type and dose of chemotherapy are the primary determinants of this risk. Radiotherapy is also a significant factor, with its impact being highly dependent on the area and method of its application [10]. **Table 1** summarizes the risk factors for treatment-related gonadotoxicity in female patients with hematological diseases.

3.1 Chemotherapy's impact on ovarian cells

Chemotherapy drugs are designed to target rapidly dividing cells, which makes the ovaries particularly vulnerable:

- *Targeting rapidly dividing cells*: The cells within maturing ovarian follicles, especially granulosa cells (which are essential for follicle nourishment) are highly susceptible to chemotherapy-induced damage due to their rapid division.

- *Observed damage*: Observed damage encompasses several forms of ovarian injury, such as apoptosis of primordial follicles, ovarian atrophy (shrinking), and cortical fibrosis (scarring of the ovarian surface).

3.2 The paradoxical depletion of resting follicles

Paradoxically, even the seemingly "resting" oocytes within primordial follicles are depleted at an accelerated rate when exposed to chemotherapy. This occurs because:

- *Unwanted activation*: During chemotherapy, primordial follicles are abnormally activated. They prematurely transition from their dormant state into a more vulnerable primary or secondary follicle state.

- *Increased vulnerability*: Once activated, these follicles become susceptible to the cytotoxic damage inflicted by chemotherapy drugs [4].

Disease	Frequently used therapies	Degree of gonadotoxic risk • Low <20% • Intermediate –20-80% • High >80%
Acute lymphoblastic leukemia	Vincristine Corticosteroids Asparaginase Anthracycline Tyrosine kinase inhibitors	Low
Acute myeloid leukemia	Cytarabine Anthracycline Fludarabine Gemtuzumab ozogamicin Tyrosine kinase inhibitors	Low
Chronic myeloid leukemia	Tyrosine kinase inhibitors	Low but potentially teratogenic
Hodgkin's lymphoma	ABVD 2 cycles escalated BEACOPP	Low
	6–8 cycles escalated BEACOPP ≥30	High
	Brentuximab Nivolumab	Unknown
Non-Hodgkin's lymphoma	6 cycles CHOP ± rituximab ≤35 6 cycles DA-EPOCH ≤35	Low
	6 cycles CHOP ≥35 6 cycles DA-EPOCH ≥35 IGEV DHAP ICE	Intermediate
Other indications	Total body RT Conditioning for HSCT (busulfan, cyclophosphamide, fludarabine, melphalan, thiotepa, BEAM)	High
	CAR T-cell therapy	Unknown but lower than BMT

Table 1.
Risk factors for treatment-related gonadotoxicity in female patients with hematological diseases.

- *Molecular pathways*: Several molecular pathways, including the phosphatidylinositol 3-kinase/PTEN/Akt pathway, are involved in this unintended activation. This pathway drives irreversible maturation, which, in a normal cycle, would lead to ovulation or atresia (degeneration). However, under chemotherapy, this activation makes them targets for destruction.

- *Concomitant effects*: Studies in mouse models have shown that cyclophosphamide, a common chemotherapy drug, triggers this pathway, inducing apoptosis in maturing follicles. The resultant reduction in inhibitory factors, typically secreted by maturing follicles, triggers an increased activation of additional primordial follicles, which ultimately leads to their extensive depletion.

3.3 Radiotoxicity to the reproductive system

The degree of radiotherapy-induced gonadotoxicity is highly contingent upon the radiation field, the total administered dose, and the method of its fractionation (division over time).

- *Direct ovarian damage*: Radiotherapy can directly harm ovarian follicles and other supporting ovarian tissues [11].

- *Damage to other reproductive organs*: Beyond the ovaries, radiation may also cause adverse effects on other reproductive organs, most notably the uterus. Such damage can compromise future pregnancy outcomes even if ovarian function is preserved.

4. Factors influencing gonadotoxicity

The risk of treatment-induced gonadotoxicity, particularly POI, in women with hematology cancer is influenced by a complex interplay of patient-specific characteristics and disease-related factors. Understanding these elements is crucial for assessing fertility risk and guiding preservation strategies [7].

4.1 Patient-related factors

The patient's age at the time of treatment stands out as the most critical factor influencing the risk of gonadotoxicity. For instance, an identical chemotherapy regimen may result in a high risk of treatment-induced amenorrhea (exceeding 80%) for patients over 40, compared to a low risk (below 20%) for those under 30 years of age [12]. Although age is the primary predictor, the influence of other anthropometric and lifestyle variables, including body mass index (BMI) and smoking status, necessitates further investigation [13].

4.2 Disease-related factors

The specific type of hematology malignancy and the chosen treatment regimen profoundly affect fertility outcomes.

4.2.1 Hodgkin lymphoma

Chemotherapy regimens for HL often include alkylating agents (e.g., MOPP, MOPP/ABV hybrid, BEACOPP), which are known for their gonadotoxic potential. Cyclophosphamide is a widely used alkylating agent with a dose-dependent gonadotoxic effect.

- *Dose-response and age*: Observations have demonstrated a distinct linear dose-response correlation between alkylating chemotherapy exposure and the incidence of Premature Ovarian Insufficiency (POI) [14, 15]. Specifically, the risk of POI increases by 23% per year of age at the time of treatment. Interestingly, the predictive effect of age on POI risk was reported to be less dominant in patients who received alkylating chemotherapy in comparison to those treated with non-alkylating regimens, despite age typically being a significant predictor [9].

- *Regimen-specific impact*: Studies on early HL treatment often show recovery of regular menstrual cycles in over 90% of women, mostly within 12 months. Conversely, the BEACOPP regimen carries a substantially elevated risk; the risk of POI increases markedly in women 30 years or older receiving this treatment, with 45% of patients reporting subsequent amenorrhea [16].

- *Ovarian reserve*: Levels of Anti-Müllerian Hormone (AMH), which serves as a marker of ovarian reserve, are noted to decline during the administration of both ABVD and BEACOPP regimens [9, 16]. One-year post-ABVD, AMH levels typically return to pre-treatment concentrations. However, age strongly influences this recovery: full recovery is common in women younger than 35, while those 35 or older often achieve only partial recovery. Overall, patients treated with BEACOPP exhibit minimal recovery in AMH levels, and the risk of POI is further compounded in those above 35 years of age [9].

4.2.2 Non-Hodgkin lymphoma and HSCT

Evidence regarding gonadotoxicity in NHL is more limited but generally points to a higher risk of permanent infertility due to the aggressive nature of treatment.

- *High prevalence of POI*: Patients undergoing HSCT for lymphoma (both HL and NHL) receive intensive conditioning regimens involving high-dose chemotherapy (including alkylating agents) with or without radiation therapy. This specific exposure results in a very high incidence of permanent POI and associated infertility (risk surpassing 80%), even when total body irradiation has not been administered. Melphalan is considered one of the most highly gonadotoxic alkylating agents. It is a key component of high-dose conditioning regimens for autologous stem cell transplantation in patients with multiple myeloma and lymphoma. Due to its potent DNA cross-linking ability, melphalan is associated with a very high rate of permanent gonadal failure in both men and women, with some studies reporting nearly 100% of female patients experiencing permanent amenorrhea after high-dose treatment [16].

- *Predictors of recovery*: The most crucial predictors of ovarian function recovery in these cases are the patient's age at the time of transplantation and the number of chemotherapy cycles received. For example, DA-EPOCH is known for its dose-adjusted nature, meaning the dose of cyclophosphamide increases with each subsequent cycle to achieve a certain degree of bone marrow suppression. Consequently, a patient who receives 6 cycles is exposed to a much higher total dose than one who receives 3 cycles, which directly correlates with a higher risk of infertility. A study of patients with primary mediastinal B-cell lymphoma treated with DA-EPOCH-R shows that although fertility recovery is more common in young women, even they can experience premature menopause or reduced ovarian reserve, which increases the long-term risk.

- *Transplantation type*: Gonadal toxicity may be exacerbated by altered immunomodulation in the alloHSCT setting compared to autologous HSCT.

- *Menstrual recovery*: Despite these severe risks, recent reports indicate higher rates of menstrual function recovery (63%) in patients with a median age of 25 years who underwent intense chemotherapy and autologous HSCT for both NHL and HL [17].

4.3 Novel immune therapies and fertility

Because these are newer therapies, large-scale, long-term studies on their fertility effects are still emerging. The current evidence is based on smaller studies, case reports, and an understanding of the drugs' mechanisms of action. As these are new therapies, large-scale, long-term studies investigating their effects on fertility are still emerging. Current evidence is therefore based on smaller studies, case reports and an understanding of how the drugs work.

- *Brentuximab vedotin (BV)*: This is an antibody-drug conjugate (ADC). The reduced gonadotoxicity is attributed to the mechanism of drug delivery directly to cancer cells, thereby minimizing systemic exposure and mitigating damage to healthy, rapidly dividing cells within the gonads [18]. However, some off-target effects and systemic release of the cytotoxic payload can still occur.

- *Immune checkpoint inhibitors*: Nivolumab/Pembrolizumab is a type of immunotherapy that works by "unleashing" the immune system to attack cancer. The primary concern for fertility with these drugs stems from their potential to cause immune-related adverse events (irAEs). In rare cases, these can affect the endocrine system by causing autoimmune inflammation of the pituitary gland (hypophysitis) or the thyroid gland. These clinical conditions may induce a disruption of the hypothalamic-pituitary-gonadal (HPG) axis, which is responsible for regulating reproductive hormones, consequently causing fertility compromise [19].

- *CAR T-cell therapy*: CAR T-cell therapy represents a significant advancement in the treatment of hematological malignancies and is becoming an increasingly vital option for young patients. Although the efficacy of the treatment in inducing remission is thoroughly established, long-term data concerning its side effects, particularly its impact on fertility, remains scarce [20]. Large, prospective studies are needed to evaluate the long-term effects of CAR T-cell therapy on male and female reproductive function. The primary gonadotoxic risk arises from the lymphodepleting chemotherapy (LDC) administered before the CAR T-cell infusion. This preparatory therapy typically includes drugs like fludarabine and cyclophosphamide. Although fludarabine and cyclophosphamide are known for their gonadotoxic effects, the doses used in CAR T-cell therapy are significantly lower than those in the myeloablative conditioning regimens used for alloHSCT. This results in a lower risk of gonadal failure. A study in the *Journal of Clinical Oncology* notes that these low-dose alkylating agents are less likely to cause irreversible gonadal damage. There are reports of reproductive function recovering in some patients after CAR T-cell therapy. Current data compiled from multiple centers confirm reports of successful pregnancies and live births subsequent to CAR T-cell therapy [21, 22]. For instance, a study documented in the journal *Blood Advances* identified multiple pregnancies resulting in five births, though only two of these involved the utilization of the patient's own retrieved oocytes [21]. Clinical cases have documented pregnancies occurring years post-therapy despite the continued presence of CAR T-cells; critically, it was observed that the CAR T-cells did not cross the placental barrier, resulting in the birth of a healthy infant [22].

In summary, a comprehensive understanding of both patient-specific characteristics (primarily age) and disease-related factors (chemotherapy regimen, dose, and the need for HSCT) is essential for accurately assessing the risk of gonadotoxicity and informing fertility preservation decisions in women with lymphoma.

5. Fertility assessment

Assessing fertility in premenopausal women is a complex process. A significant challenge, affecting not only those who have undergone chemo/radiotherapy, is POI. It has been shown that POI can occur even when the menstrual cycle returns after treatment, primarily due to the depletion of primordial follicles. It is crucial to understand that amenorhea does not automatically mean infertility. Conversely, women whose menstrual cycles resume may still experience compromised fertility.

The state of ovarian reserve, as determined by the number of follicles containing oocytes, provides reliable information regarding fertility. It is hypothesized that AMH levels and antral follicle count (AFC), as determined by transvaginal ultrasound, offer superior diagnostic accuracy compared with conventional markers of female fertility, including estradiol, follicle-stimulating hormone (FSH), luteinizing hormone (LH), and menstrual cycle analysis. While traditional markers like FSH and estradiol are used to assess ovarian reserve, they are unreliable in the context of cancer treatment due to transient hormonal suppression. Chemotherapy administration may suppress the hypothalamic-pituitary-ovarian axis, resulting in spuriously low levels of FSH and estradiol that fail to accurately represent the long-term status of the ovarian follicle pool [4]. AMH concentration directly correlates with the size of the primordial follicle pool. Research in young cancer survivors has demonstrated that a considerable post-chemotherapy decrease in AMH levels is a reliable predictor of subsequent long-term ovarian damage and POI Research in young cancer survivors has demonstrated that a considerable post-chemotherapy decrease in AMH levels is a reliable predictor of subsequent long-term ovarian damage and POI [23]. A sonographic count of follicles, AFC offers a direct morphological assessment of the ovarian reserve. Studies indicate that a reduction in AFC following chemotherapy strongly correlates with long-term ovarian dysfunction and infertility [24].

ESHRE advocates for a robust assessment of ovarian reserve, predominantly via AMH measurement, prior to gonadotoxic treatment initiation, citing the strong correlation of AMH with long-term reproductive outcomes, which stands in contrast to the transient and non-representative nature of FSH and estradiol levels. When integrated with patient age and specific treatment plan parameters (i.e., type and dose), this assessment facilitates a more accurate forecast of post-treatment ovarian function recovery and the individual risk of POI development [25].

6. Ovarian stimulation for fertility preservation in hematological malignancies: Challenges and recommendations

Ovarian stimulation and egg retrieval for fertility preservation in women with hematological cancers present a unique set of challenges. This procedure is generally considered only for women with no obvious contraindications for ovarian stimulation or egg collection.

6.1 Navigating time constraints and medical risks

A significant hurdle is the time-sensitive nature of cancer treatment. Typically, around two weeks are needed to retrieve enough eggs. This timeframe often clashes with the urgent need to start anticancer therapy, especially given the rapid progression of hematological diseases. Patients also face risks like thrombosis, hemorrhage, and infections due to low platelet (thrombocytopenia) and white blood cell (leukocytopenia) counts, which can complicate fertility preservation procedures.

6.2 Managing the risk of ovarian hyperstimulation syndrome (OHSS)

Ovarian Hyperstimulation Syndrome (OHSS) is a potential concern for all patients undergoing ovarian stimulation, particularly young women or those expected to produce many eggs. Large studies show that the risk of OHSS increases when more than 15 oocytes are collected. Nevertheless, no elevated risks have been documented in patients with either benign or malignant diseases who underwent ovarian stimulation for cryopreservation and achieved an average retrieval of 10–12 oocytes [25]. Still, more extensive multicenter international data are needed for precise risk estimates in cancer patients.

6.3 Recommended protocols for oncohematological patients

For patients with oncohematological diseases, the GnRH antagonist protocol for Controlled Ovarian Stimulation (COS) is generally recommended. This protocol is favored due to its:

- *Feasibility in urgent situations*: It allows for quicker initiation.
- *Short duration*: Minimizing delays to cancer treatment.
- *Favorable safety profile*: Helping to mitigate risks.

This methodology provides advantages such as a reduced duration of stimulation. Furthermore, it permits the use of a GnRH agonist to trigger oocyte maturation in high-responder patients, thereby mitigating the risk of Ovarian Hyperstimulation Syndrome (OHSS) [25].

Additionally, for urgent fertility preservation cycles, ovarian stimulation with a random start is an option, meaning it does not have to begin at a specific point in the menstrual cycle. If chemotherapy initiation allows multiple stimulation cycles or even double stimulation within the same cycle (DuoStim) can be performed in cases of low response to increase the number of available eggs. DuoStim leverages the fact that follicles can be recruited for growth at different times in the menstrual cycle, not just during the follicular phase [26]. Stimulating the ovaries twice within a single cycle enables the harvesting of mature oocytes from two distinct follicular cohorts, consequently doubling the potential yield of retrieved oocytes [27]. This is a critical advantage for patients with limited time before starting gonadotoxic therapy. Evidence from key studies supports its feasibility and efficacy. Research in oncology patients has demonstrated that DuoStim can yield a higher number of mature oocytes compared to a single conventional stimulation cycle. Studies specifically in poor responders undergoing fertility preservation have shown that the number of oocytes and embryos retrieved in the luteal phase stimulation is comparable to or better than that from the follicular phase, confirming its effectiveness. Careful timing is crucial. The luteal phase stimulation can be initiated as soon as 2–5 days after the first oocyte retrieval. This rapid sequencing allows the entire process to be completed in a condensed period, making it suitable for patients needing to start cancer treatment promptly [27]. The use of random-start stimulation protocols in conjunction with DuoStim further enhances its flexibility.

7. Fertility preserving procedures

Fertility preserving options in young women with hematological malignancies could be divided into established, debatable, and experimental. Nevertheless, each of those options has both advantages and disadvantages and may not be feasible for all patients.

7.1 Established options

7.1.1 Oocyte/embryo cryopreservation

The gold standard for fertility preservation in women is cryopreservation of oocytes or embryos after COCs lasting 10–14 days. It is important to note that there are often limitations related to the specificity of the hematological neoplasias and extremely reduced time frame represents an important issue. These factors include the need to initiate antitumour therapy on an emergency basis, severe cytopenias, and coagulation disorders that make delaying treatment and oocytes aspiration risky. It is important to note that the method is not suitable for prepubertal girls. The efficacy of the procedure depends on several factors, including the age of the woman undergoing the procedure (given the increasing incidence of aneuploidy with age), the method of cryopreservation employed (specifically, whether slow freezing or ventilation is used), and the presence of any concomitant endocrine or gynecological pathology. A US-based study indicated that the cumulative pregnancy rate post-embryo transfer was comparable between cancer patients and age-matched controls, with rates of 37% and 43%, respectively [5]. Oocyte cryopreservation is an appropriate procedure for women without a partner and in countries that have legal restrictions on embryo storage.

Embryo freezing requires prior ovarian stimulation, mature oocyte retrieval, and sperm for IVF. Therefore, it is not suitable for prepubertal girls due to inactive hypothalamic-pituitary-ovarian (HPO) axis and not suitable for single women refusing sperm donation for any reason. The established cryostorage duration for gametes (eggs and sperm) and embryos is 10 years, though the possibility of extended storage is subject to variation based on local and national regulatory frameworks [25]. Pregnancy rates subsequent to embryo cryopreservation in women are comparable to those observed in women undergoing treatment for infertility in other indications.

7.2 Debatable options

7.2.1 Gonadotropin-releasing hormone agonists (GnRHa)

GnRHa provide protection to the ovary during chemotherapy by suppressing ovarian function. The mechanism of action of GnRHa is unclear, and the effect remains controversial. The positive effect of agonists has been demonstrated in breast cancer patients. Most studies evaluating the protective role of GnRHa have included patients with heterogeneous characteristics, defined different endpoints, and various types, doses and regimens of the drugs were used. A recent meta-analysis reported a reduced rate of persistent amenorrhea when GnRHa was co-administered with chemotherapy (RR 0.60, 95% CI 0.45–0.79) [28]. The protective effect was more pronounced with low/moderate intensity HT. Subgroup analysis of women with lymphoma revealed that concomitant use of GnRHa did not result in a reduction in the likelihood of POF/amenorrhea (RR 0.70; 95% CI: 0.45–0.79) or spontaneous pregnancy (RR 1.13, 95% CI: 0.66–1.93). Similar outcomes were identified in a 2019 Cochrane review, which demonstrated an increased rate of menstrual function recovery during a follow-up period of up to 12 months (RR 1.60, 95% CI 1.14–2.24) [29]. Furthermore, GnRHa is not an appropriate option in prepubertal girls. The administration of GnRHa remains an unproven method of fertility protection in patients with malignant hematological diseases. GnRH agonists should not be routinely offered as an option to protect ovarian function and an equivalent or alternative to preserve fertility. They may be offered after cryopreservation techniques have been implemented or when they are not feasible. An additional medical benefit of administering GnRH agonists during chemotherapy is prevention of heavy menstrual bleeding which may be of value for patients receiving chemotherapy regimens with high bone marrow toxicity. Observational data suggest that oral contraceptives may also reduce the risk of POI, but no proper randomized studies have demonstrated their effect.

7.2.2 Oophoropexy

Oophoropexy is the surgical relocation of the ovaries to protect them from pelvic radiotherapy, typically used for pelvic malignancies like HL. Crucially, the procedure offers no protection against chemotherapy-induced gonadotoxicity. Therefore, it is impractical to perform oophoropexy on patients scheduled to receive combined (concomitant) chemotherapy.

7.2.3 Gonadal shielding

Gonadal shielding offers some protection for the ovaries, particularly for young patients. However, like oophoropexy, it cannot prevent damage to the ovaries caused by chemotherapy. Therefore, its use is limited when chemotherapy is part of the treatment plan.

7.2.4 Fractionated radiotherapy

To minimize gonadotoxicity and gonadal damage, the fractionation of radiotherapy doses should be attempted whenever possible.

7.2.5 Ovarian tissue cryopreservation (OTC)

For some women with hematological disease, cryopreservation of ovarian tissue may be the only option. It is recommended for patients undergoing moderate/high-risk gonadotoxic treatment when oocyte/embryo cryopreservation is not feasible, or at the patient's preference. One of the major advantages of OTC compared to oocyte/embryo cryopreservation is the possibility to perform the procedure after starting chemotherapy treatment without hormonal stimulation. Patients may benefit from a first line regimen before OTC or can be referred to for OTC before consolidation therapy such as conditioning regimen for HSCT or after a limited response to low gonadotoxic regimen such as standard ABVD (doxorubicin, bleomycin, vinblastine, dacarbazine) for Hodgkin lymphoma [16]. The interval between OTC and the last chemotherapy treatment must be taken into consideration for the evaluation of ovarian reserve testing. Either an ovarian cortex biopsy (the location of the primordial follicle pool) or one whole ovary can be retrieved at any time during the menstrual cycle and the cortex cryopreserved for future restoration of ovarian function. Laparoscopy remains the predominant technique for tissue collection. The procedure is advantageous as it preserves both fertility and endogenous hormonal secretion, thereby conferring beneficial effects on cardiovascular and bone health, as well as sexual function [30]. It is challenging because of the risk of infection and bleeding, and the possibility of contaminating the tissue with malignant cells. Cryopreservation of ovarian tissue is not appropriate for patients with low ovarian reserve (AMH <0.5 ng/ml and/or AFC <5) or for elderly patients. The effectiveness of the procedure for women over 36 years of age is questionable. Reports of ovarian autotransplantation in Hodgkin's lymphoma patients exceed 100 cases, with no documented instances of disease relapse [16]. Reports in non-Hodgkin lymphoma are more limited. The first baby born after the transplantation of cryopreserved ovarian tissue in a patient with leukemia was in 2018. This is the only option for preserving fertility in prepubertal girls. The primary limitation of this technique stems from the risk of tumor cell contamination within the ovarian tissue graft, a concern particularly relevant in malignancies characterized by hematologic dissemination. The risk level is highest for leukemia patients, followed by non-Hodgkin's lymphoma, while the probability is markedly lower for solid tumors and Hodgkin's lymphoma [23].

7.3 Future prospects

7.3.1 Artificial ovaries

The artificial ovary concept centers on the development of a biocompatible scaffold engineered to support the growth and subsequent maturation of primordial follicles isolated from the patient's own ovarian tissue [31]. The primary driver for developing this approach is the need to circumvent a critical risk in hematological malignancies (such as leukemia) and other cancers with a high propensity for ovarian metastasis: the potential for inadvertently re-implanting malignant cells along with the ovarian tissue [32]. Recent preclinical studies, particularly in animal models, have demonstrated the feasibility of this technology. While the results are promising, there are major hurdles to overcome before clinical application. Key challenges include ensuring the long-term viability of the follicles, achieving full oocyte maturation, and replicating the complex hormonal and vascular environment of a natural ovary [33, 34]. Currently, no clinical trials of a fully functional artificial ovary are underway, and the technology remains in the experimental research phase.

7.3.2 In vitro *follicle maturation (IVF-M) and stem cells*

In vitro follicle maturation (IVF-M) is the process of growing immature follicles in a lab setting to the stage where they can produce mature, fertilizable eggs [32]. This is closely related to stem cell technologies, as both aim to create viable gametes outside the body, bypassing the need for whole-ovary transplantation [35, 36]. Researchers are exploring the use of oogonial stem cells (OSCs) and other adult stem cells, such as those from the bone marrow, to regenerate gonadal function. Research involving murine models has demonstrated that the transplantation of these stem cells can successfully restore oogenesis, leading, in some cases, to the birth of live offspring. This methodology offers a potential pathway for fertility restoration in patients who were unable to undergo tissue banking prior to therapeutic intervention [36]. While these studies are exciting, they are still in early preclinical stages and are not yet ready for human application. The primary challenge is replicating the intricate cellular interactions and signaling pathways required for full human oocyte maturation in a lab setting. The risk of cancer recurrence from re-injecting even small numbers of stem cells remains a significant concern and requires extensive research to ensure safety. Therefore, these are considered "emerging" technologies and are not yet a standard clinical option for patients.

8. Outside fertility preservation

If fertility preservation options are rejected, contraindicated, infeasible, unavailable, or unsuccessful, adoption and third-party reproduction (egg donation, embryo donation, and surrogacy) can be offered as family-building alternatives. If third-party reproduction services are not available or not legally allowed in a country, patients may travel abroad to obtain them.

9. How long should patients be in remission?

Although conceiving after cancer treatment does not increase the risk of cancer recurrence, it is still unknown whether short intervals between treatment and conception might cause poor pregnancy outcomes. It is recommended that any attempt to conceive through assisted reproduction be initiated a minimum of two years after complete remission of the hematological disease has been achieved. The two-year timeframe is based on a few key clinical and biological considerations:

- *Highest relapse risk*: For many cancer types, especially hematological malignancies like lymphoma and leukemia, the highest risk of disease recurrence is within the first one to two years after achieving complete remission. A significant portion of relapses occur during this period, and a new pregnancy could complicate or delay essential cancer treatment, potentially jeopardizing the patient's life.

- *Maternal and fetal safety*: The occurrence of cancer relapse during pregnancy requires navigating complex decisions concerning the continuation of the gestation in balance with the necessity of resuming aggressive anticancer treatment [37, 38]. This could lead to poor pregnancy outcomes. Therefore, waiting until the patient is past this critical relapse window significantly reduces this risk.

- *Physical and emotional recovery*: Cancer treatment, particularly chemotherapy, can be physically and emotionally taxing. The two-year waiting period allows the body to recover, replenish its reserves, and for the patient to mentally and emotionally prepare for a healthy pregnancy.

Consequently, leading oncology and fertility organizations, including the European Society for Medical Oncology (ESMO) and the American Society of Clinical Oncology (ASCO) [39, 40], advise a minimum waiting period of two years following complete remission. It is important to note that this is a general guideline. The final decision should be based on an individualized risk assessment, taking into account the specific type of cancer, stage, prognosis, and the patient's overall health. For some cancers with a very low risk of early relapse, a shorter waiting period might be considered after a thorough discussion between the patient, their oncohematologist, and the fertility specialist. This ensures a balance between fertility goals and long-term survival.

10. Conclusion

Fertility preservation represents a major issue for young women suffering from malignant hematological diseases. The impact of hematological neoplasia on fertility varies and depends on several factors. The most important factors are the nature of the disease, the regimen and dose of chemotherapeutic medication administered, the patient's age, and AMH levels. The risk of gonadotoxicity should be assessed for all patients undergoing gonadotoxic treatment. Despite any concomitant complications or the need for prompt antitumor therapy, adequate replacement therapy, anti-infective prophylaxis, and timely consultation with a reproductive specialist can provide this opportunity. Effective communication and collaboration between the treating hematologist, the reproductive specialist, and the patient are pivotal to the successful completion of the process. Unfortunately, reports indicate that 50% of patients state they have not engaged in a discussion regarding fertility issues with their primary treating physician [41].

Take-home messages

- The risk of gonadotoxicity should be assessed in every patient undergoing gonadotoxic therapy.
- Any patient with a hematologic malignancy should be consulted by a reproductive specialist.
- Fertility preservation in patients with hematologic neoplasia is possible after careful risk/benefit assessment.
- The gold standard for fertility preservation in hematologic oncology patients is oocyte/embryo cryopreservation after a short protocol COS.
- Cryopreservation of ovarian tissue is possible but under certain conditions.
- The administration of GnRHa remains an unproven method of fertility protection in patients with hematologic malignancies. GnRH agonists should not be routinely offered as an option to protect ovarian function and an equivalent or alternative to fertility preservation. They may be offered after cryopreservation techniques have been implemented or when they are not possible.

Conflict of interest

The authors declare no conflict of interest.

Author details

Georgi Stamenov[1] and Kameliya Kostadinova[2]*

1 Nadezhda Women's Health Hospital Obstetrics and Gynecology Department, Sofia, Bulgaria

2 Specialized Hospital for Active Treatment of Hematological Diseases, Sofia, Bulgaria

*Address all correspondence to: vomodo@abv.bg

References

[1] National Institutes of Health. Cancer Stat Facts: Leukemia — Acute Lymphocytic Leukemia (ALL). n.d. Available from: https://seer.cancer.gov/statfacts/html/alyl.html

[2] Cusatis R et al. Current trends and outcomes in cellular therapy activity in the United States, including prospective patient-reported outcomes data collection in the Center for International Blood and Marrow Transplant Research registry. Transplantation and Cellular Therapy. 2024;**30**(9):917.e1-917.e12. DOI: 10.1016/j.jtct.2024.06.021

[3] Meirow D, Biederman H, Anderson RA, Wallace WH. Toxicity of chemotherapy and radiation on female reproduction. Clinical Obstetrics and Gynecology. 2010;**53**(4):727-739

[4] Shimoji S, Hashimoto D, Tsujigiwa H, Miyawaki K, Kato K, Takahashi S, et al. Graft-versus-host disease targets ovary and causes female infertility in mice. Blood. 2017;**129**(9):1216-1225

[5] Chow EJ, Stratton KL, Leisenring WM, et al. Pregnancy after chemotherapy in male and female survivors of childhood cancer treated between 1970 and 1999: A report from the childhood cancer survivor study cohort. Lancet Oncology. 2016;**17**(5):567-576

[6] Carter A, Robison LL, Francisco L, et al. Prevalence of conception and pregnancy outcomes after hematopoietic cell transplantation: Report from the bone marrow transplant survivor study. Bone Marrow Transplantation. 2006;**37**(11):1023-1029

[7] Faddy MJ, Gosden RG, Gougeon A, Richardson SJ, Nelson JF. Accelerated disappearance of ovarian follicles in mid-life: Implications for forecasting menopause. Human Reproduction. 1992;**7**(10):1342-1346

[8] Lee SJ et al. American Society of Clinical Oncology recommendations on fertility preservation in cancer patients. Journal of Clinical Oncology. 2006;**24**(18):2917-2931. DOI: 10.1200/JCO.2006.06.5888

[9] Wallace WH, Thomson AB, Saran F, Kelsey TW. Predicting age of ovarian failure after radiation to a field that includes the ovaries. International Journal of Radiation Oncology Biology Physics. 2005;**62**(3):738-744

[10] Ruddy KJ et al. Chemotherapy-related amenorrhea after adjuvant paclitaxel-trastuzumab (APT trial). Breast Cancer Research and Treatment. 2015;**151**(3):589-596. DOI: 10.1007/s10549-015-3426-z

[11] Abusief ME et al. Relationship between reproductive history, anthropometrics, lifestyle factors, and the likelihood of persistent chemotherapy-related amenorrhea in women with premenopausal breast cancer. Fertility and Sterility. 2012;**97**(1):154-159. DOI: 10.1016/j.fertnstert.2011.10.009

[12] van der Kaaij MA et al. Premature ovarian failure and fertility in long-term survivors of Hodgkin's lymphoma: A European Organisation for Research and Treatment of Cancer Lymphoma Group and Groupe d'Etude des Lymphomes de l'Adulte cohort study. Journal of Clinical Oncology. 2012;**30**(3):291-299. DOI: 10.1200/JCO.2011.37.1989

[13] Behringer K et al. Gonadal function and fertility in survivors after Hodgkin

lymphoma treatment within the German Hodgkin Study Group HD13 to HD15 trials. Journal of Clinical Oncology. 2013;**31**(2):231-239. DOI: 10.1200/JCO.2012.44.3721

[14] Anderson RA et al. Determinants of ovarian function after response-adapted therapy in patients with advanced Hodgkin's lymphoma. Lancet Oncology. 2018;**19**(10):1328-1337

[15] Loren AW, Senapati S. Fertility preservation in patients with hematologic malignancies. Blood. 2019;**134**(9):746-760. DOI: 10.1182/blood.2018846790

[16] Himpe J, Lammerant S, Van den Bergh L, Lapeire L, De Roo C. The impact of systemic oncological treatments on the fertility of adolescents and young adults—A systematic review. Life (Basel). 2023;**13**(5):1209. DOI: 10.3390/life13051209

[17] Küçük M, Bolaman AZ, Yavaşoğlu I, Kadıköylü G. Fertility-preserving treatment options in patients with malignant hematological diseases. Turkish Journal of Haematology. 2012;**29**(3):207-216. DOI: 10.5505/tjh.2012.72681

[18] Silvestris E et al. Fertility preservation in the era of immuno-oncology: Lights and shadows. Journal of Personalized Medicine. 2024;**14**(4):431. DOI: 10.3390/jpm14040431

[19] Ligon JA et al. Fertility and CAR T-cells: Current practice and future directions. Transplantation and Cellular Therapy. 2022;**28**(9):605.e1-605.e8. DOI: 10.1016/j.jtct.2022.06.002

[20] Ligon J, Logan N, Li G. Fertility outcomes following CAR T-cell therapy: Results from a patient-facing survey. Transplantation and Cellular Therapy. n.d.;**32S**:353

[21] Canty EA et al. First reported case of a spontaneous and healthy pregnancy in a woman with persistent CAR T-cells 5 years after treatment for diffuse large B-cell lymphoma. Journal for Immunotherapy of Cancer. 2025;**13**(4):e011092. DOI: 10.1136/jitc-2024-011092

[22] Anderson RA et al. Anti-Müllerian hormone as a marker of ovarian reserve and premature ovarian insufficiency in children and women with cancer: A systematic review. Human Reproduction Update. 2022;**28**(3):417-434. DOI: 10.1093/humupd/dmac004

[23] Gracia CR et al. Impact of cancer therapies on ovarian reserve. Fertility and Sterility. 2012;**97**(1):134-40.e1. DOI: 10.1016/j.fertnstert.2011.10.040

[24] The ESHRE Guideline Group on Female Fertility Preservation et al. ESHRE guideline: Female fertility preservation. Human Reproduction Open. 2020;**2020**(4):hoaa052. DOI: 10.1093/hropen/hoaa052

[25] Liu C, Jiang H, Zhang W, Yin H. Double ovarian stimulation during the follicular and luteal phase in women ≥38 years: A retrospective case-control study. Reproductive Biomedicine Online. 2017;**35**(6):678-684. DOI: 10.1016/j.rbmo.2017.08.019

[26] Gica C et al. Double ovarian stimulation in the same ovarian cycle. Maedica (Bucur). 2021;**16**(1):102-106. DOI: 10.26574/maedica.2020.16.1.97

[27] Lambertini M et al. Gonadotropin-releasing hormone agonists during chemotherapy for preservation of ovarian function and fertility in premenopausal patients with early breast cancer: A systematic review and meta-analysis. Journal of Clinical Oncology. 2018;**36**(19):1981-1990. DOI: 10.1200/JCO.2018.78.0858

[28] Chen H, Xiao L, Li J, Cui L, Huang W. Adjuvant gonadotropin-releasing hormone analogues for the prevention of chemotherapy-induced premature ovarian failure in premenopausal women. Cochrane Database of Systematic Reviews. 2019;**3**(3):CD008018. DOI: 10.1002/14651858.CD008018.pub3

[29] Dolmans MM, Luyckx V, Donnez J, Stoop D, Ammon Richard P. Safety of ovarian tissue transplantation in cancer patients. ISRN Obstetrics and Gynecology. 2012;**2012**:495142. DOI: 10.1155/2012/495142

[30] Amorim CA, Shikanov A. The artificial ovary: Current status and future perspectives. Future Oncology. 2016;**12**(20):2323-2332

[31] Chiti MC et al. A novel fibrin-based artificial ovary prototype resembling human ovarian tissue in terms of architecture and rigidity. Journal of Assisted Reproduction and Genetics. 2018;**35**(1):41-48

[32] Soares M et al. Eliminating malignant cells from cryopreserved ovarian tissue is possible in leukaemia patients. British Journal of Haematology. 2017;**178**(2):231-239

[33] Laronda MM et al. A bioprosthetic ovary created using 3D printed microporous scaffolds restores ovarian function in sterilized mice. Nature Communications. 2017;**8**:15261. DOI: 10.1038/ncomms15261

[34] Nair R, Kasturi M, Mathur V, Seetharam RN, Vasanthan KS. Strategies for developing 3D printed ovarian model for restoring fertility. Clinical and Translational Science. 2024;**17**(7):e13863. DOI: 10.1111/cts.13863

[35] Dolmans MM, Amorim CA. Fertility preservation: Construction and use of artificial ovaries. Reproduction. 2019;**158**(5):F15-F25. DOI: 10.1530/REP-18-0536

[36] Kim JM, Kim S, Lee S. Role of stem cells in the ovarian tissue cryopreservation and transplantation for fertility preservation. International Journal of Molecular Sciences. 2021;**22**(22):12482. DOI: 10.3390/ijms222212482

[37] Azim HA Jr et al. Safety of pregnancy following breast cancer diagnosis: A meta-analysis of 14 studies. European Journal of Cancer. 2011;**47**(1):74-83. DOI: 10.1016/j.ejca.2010.09.007

[38] Dolmans MM, Masciangelo R. Construction and use of artificial ovaries in fertility preservation. Reproduction. 2018;**158**(5):R145-R154

[39] Peccatori FA et al. Cancer, fertility and pregnancy: ESMO clinical practice guidelines. Annals of Oncology. 2013;**24**(suppl 6):vi160-vi170

[40] Oktay K et al. Fertility preservation in patients with cancer: ASCO clinical practice guideline update. Journal of Clinical Oncology. 2018;**36**(16):1999-2009

[41] American Society of Clinical Oncology. Only Half of Young Adults with cancer Are Told of Fertility Preservation Options by their Providers. The ASCO Post; 2025. Available from: https://ascopost.com/issues/february-25-2025/only-half-of-young-adults-with-cancer-are-told-of-fertility-preservation-options-by-their-providers/

Chapter 6

Epigenetic Stability and Genomic Integrity in Fertility Preservation: Insights from Genetic and Reproductive Technologies

Songlin Zhang, Chenglu Wang, Leixiang Yang, Min Zheng, Xiaohua Tang and Xiaopan Chen

Abstract

Fertility preservation techniques—particularly cryopreservation and thawing—are essential in reproductive medicine for safeguarding the reproductive potential of individuals facing medical or elective fertility challenges. However, these interventions expose gametes (oocytes and sperm), embryos, and reproductive tissues to physical and molecular stress, potentially compromising both epigenetic stability and genomic integrity. This chapter reviews current knowledge on the maintenance and disruption of DNA methylation patterns, histone modifications, chromatin structure, and non-coding RNA (ncRNA) profiles during storage, alongside potential alterations in nuclear and mitochondrial genomes that may influence developmental competence and transgenerational health. We summarize technological advances in genetic and assisted reproductive technologies, evaluate their impact on molecular integrity, and outline strategies to mitigate damage. Emphasis is placed on the need for standardized protocols, comprehensive genomic and epigenomic assessment, and long-term monitoring to ensure the safety and efficacy of fertility preservation.

Keywords: fertility preservation, cryopreservation, epigenetic stability, genomic integrity, mitochondrial DNA, histone modification

1. Introduction

Fertility preservation has become an integral component of modern reproductive medicine, providing a crucial option for individuals undergoing gonadotoxic treatments, experiencing age-related fertility decline, suffering from autoimmune diseases, or choosing to delay childbearing for personal or social reasons [1, 2]. Among the various existing strategies, cryopreservation, especially oocyte cryopreservation, has emerged as the most widely used and technologically mature method. In the United States alone, the number of oocyte cryopreservation cycles performed in 2021 exceeded 24,000, showing a

IntechOpen

substantial increase compared to previous years and highlighting its central role in fertility preservation [3]. This global trend has been fueled by improved vitrification protocols, expanded clinical indications, and rising public awareness. The cryopreservation of gametes, embryos, and gonadal tissues has revolutionized assisted reproductive technologies (ART), enabling individuals to preserve reproductive potential in both medical and elective contexts [4]. However, as the clinical use of cryopreserved materials becomes more widespread, growing attention is being directed toward their long-term safety, particularly concerning epigenetic fidelity, genomic integrity, and potential transgenerational effects on offspring [5].

Epigenetics refers to reversible and heritable changes in gene expression that occur independently of alterations to the underlying DNA sequence and are influenced by both internal and external factors [6]. It encompasses a wide range of molecular mechanisms, including DNA methylation, histone modifications, non-coding RNAs (ncRNAs), and chromatin remodeling [7]. These processes play essential roles during germ cell specification, gametogenesis, and early embryonic development. Through chemical modifications of the genome, epigenetic mechanisms regulate gene accessibility and activity, guiding cell differentiation, parental imprinting, cell-type-specific gene expression, X-chromosome inactivation, and the preservation of genomic structure and stability [8–10].

Genomic integrity, on the other hand, refers to the maintenance of both the structural and functional stability of nuclear DNA (nDNA) and mitochondrial DNA (mtDNA), ensuring protection against mutations, double-strand breaks (DSBs), chromosomal aberrations, and oxidative stress. Although DNA is often regarded as chemically stable, it is inherently a dynamic molecule that remains vulnerable to a wide range of endogenous and exogenous insults [11]. During cryopreservation—most commonly involving ultra-low temperature storage in liquid nitrogen (−196°C)—biological samples are subjected to substantial physicochemical stress, including osmotic fluctuations, intracellular ice crystal formation, and the accumulation of reactive oxygen species (ROS), all of which can compromise genomic stability [12]. Notably, hyperosmotic stress has been shown to induce chromosomal abnormalities and elevate the frequency of sister chromatid exchanges, potentially via mechanisms such as ionic imbalance, macromolecular crowding, excessive ROS generation, and alterations in chromatin architecture [13]. These stressors may increase mechanical strain on DNA or enhance its accessibility to nucleases, thereby promoting DSB formation. Mitochondrial DNA, which lacks protective histones and resides close to the electron transport chain, is particularly susceptible to oxidative damage during cryopreservation, leading to point mutations, large-scale deletions, and impaired mitochondrial function [14].

This chapter aims to provide a comprehensive overview of how fertility preservation impacts epigenetic modifications and genomic architecture within gametes, embryos, and preserved reproductive tissues. We explore how advances in reproductive and genetic technologies have enhanced our ability to monitor, understand, and mitigate the molecular alterations induced by cryopreservation, particularly changes affecting DNA methylation patterns, histone landscapes, chromatin organization, and mitochondrial genome integrity. Current strategies designed to minimize such molecular damage are highlighted, alongside a discussion of ethical considerations and the pressing need for standardized protocols and long-term follow-up studies. By integrating perspectives from epigenetics and reproductive genetics, this chapter outlines future directions to better understand transgenerational consequences and improve clinical outcomes in fertility preservation.

2. Epigenetic mechanisms in embryos and gametes

Epigenetic reprogramming is a vital process during human gametogenesis and early embryogenesis, orchestrating a genome-wide epigenome reset to secure developmental potential [8]. This tightly regulated process governs DNA methylation, histone post-translational modifications (PTMs), and chromatin reorganization, facilitating the erasure of parental epigenetic imprints and the establishment of totipotent and pluripotent states [15, 16]. Mice are essential models for unraveling human epigenetic mechanisms, offering critical insights into the molecular foundations of reprogramming. Disruptions in this process can result in reproductive dysfunction, imprinting disorders such as Beckwith-Wiedemann syndrome and Angelman syndrome, and developmental abnormalities [17, 18].

Following human embryo implantation, primordial germ cells (PGCs) differentiate from epiblast cells, exhibiting an epigenetic state similar to neighboring somatic-fated cells, retaining stable DNA methylation and X-chromosome inactivation, which pose barriers to achieving totipotency [19–21]. Early PGC development requires extensive reprogramming to overcome these barriers. The first significant chromatin changes include the loss of H3K9me2 around Week 4 and a global increase in H3K27me3 by Week 5 (**Figure 1A**) [22–24]. Both are repressive modifications; the increase in H3K27me3 may compensate for the loss of H3K9me2 to maintain

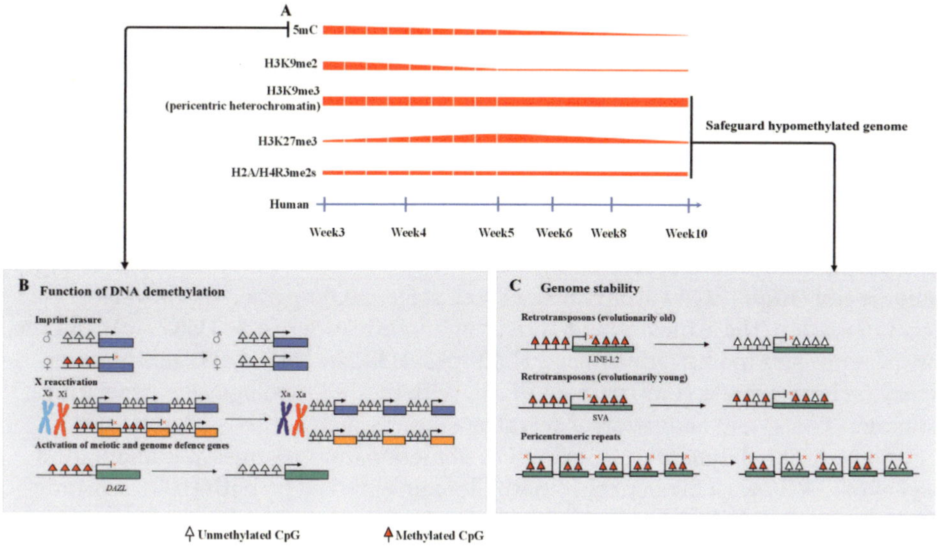

Figure 1.
Epigenetic reprogramming in human PGCs. (A) During early development, human primordial germ cells (hPGCs) undergo genome-wide DNA demethylation from Week 3 to Week 10, accompanied by dynamic changes in chromatin modifications. Levels of H3K9me2 decrease, supporting DNA demethylation, while H3K27me3 is transiently enriched during migration and later declines. H3K9me3 persists at pericentric heterochromatin, and H2A/H4R3me2s levels remain stable. (B) DNA demethylation in hPGCs erases parental imprints, facilitating germ cell development. Imprinting control regions (ICRs) are demethylated and subsequently re-established in a sex-specific manner. In female hPGCs, the inactive X chromosome is reactivated through the loss of DNA methylation and H3K27me3. Promoters of germline-specific genes, typically methylated and silenced in somatic cells, become demethylated, enabling their expression (e.g., DAZL*). (C) Despite global demethylation, transposable elements remain repressed. Evolutionarily older elements (e.g., LINE-L2) and younger ones (e.g., SVA) are silenced through histone modifications and partial DNA methylation at specific sites, maintaining genome stability during reprogramming.*

transcriptional silencing [25]. In female PGCs, H3K27me3 enrichment on the inactive X chromosome gradually decreases, reflecting X-chromosome reactivation (**Figure 1B**) [26].

During the migratory phase, PGCs acquire transcriptional and epigenetic features resembling embryonic stem (ES) cells and can give rise to embryonic germ (EG) cells in vitro [27, 28]. At this stage, H2A/H4R3me2s levels increase, catalyzed by PRMT5, supporting unipotency and suppressing somatic differentiation programs [29, 30]. Genome-wide DNA methylation (5mC) begins to decline around Week 3, primarily due to BLIMP1- and PRDM14-mediated repression of Dnmt3a, Dnmt3b, and Uhrf1 [31], possibly with contributions from GLP downregulation (**Figure 1A**) [32]. Most genomic regions—including transposable elements, imprinted loci, and single-copy genes—retain CpG methylation until Week 5, with only partial conversion of 5mC to 5-hydroxymethylcytosine (5hmC) [32, 33]. UHRF2, upregulated during PGC specification, may maintain residual 5mC by binding hemi-methylated DNA associated with H3K9me3 [34, 35].

Upon entering the genital ridges, PGCs undergo rapid, likely active, genome-wide DNA demethylation, predominantly occurring in the G2 phase. By Week 10, methylation is almost completely erased, including parental imprints and CpG methylation at promoters of germline-specific genes [24, 36]. This stage, termed the "epigenomic nadir," is accompanied by chromatin remodeling, including transient reorganization of linker histone H1, dynamic changes in H3K27me3 and H3K9me3, and stable alterations in H3K9ac and H2A/H4R3me2s (**Figure 1A**) [24]. Some retrotransposons, such as IAP elements, partially evade demethylation [37]. Research suggests that 5mC clearance in PGCs may involve a biphasic yet potentially continuous process. Compared to zygotic reprogramming, PGC reprogramming is more extensive, as the latter retains methylation at multiple loci, imprinted regions, and Polycomb-mediated chromatin modifications [38].

After fertilization, a second wave of reprogramming initiates the transition from the parental to the zygotic genome. The paternal genome undergoes rapid TET3-dependent active demethylation, while the maternal genome is passively demethylated during replication, protected by factors such as STELLA [39]. In humans, zygotic genome activation (ZGA) occurs at the 8-cell stage, accompanied by chromatin decondensation, the acquisition of activating modifications (e.g., H3K27ac), and the loss of repressive modifications (e.g., H3K9me3, H3K27me3) [16, 39]. Chromatin structure becomes less compartmentalized, with relaxed topologically associating domains (TADs) and activation of retrotransposons such as LINE-L2, influencing transcriptional dynamics (**Figure 1C**). Remethylation resumes at implantation via DNMT3A/B, with bivalent chromatin domains marked by both H3K4me3 and H3K27me3 priming lineage-specific genes.

In humans, genome-wide demethylation is mediated by TET1/2/3, which oxidize 5mC to 5hmC, facilitating both passive and active demethylation [40]. Incomplete demethylation in human PGCs results in residual methylation in mature gametes, a key species-specific difference. During oogenesis, de novo DNA methylation preferentially occurs in actively transcribed regions, guided by H3K36me3 and mediated by the DNMT3A/3 L complex to establish maternal imprints [40, 41]. During spermatogenesis, most histones are replaced by protamines, but retained histones at regulatory sites carry H3K4me3 and H3K27me3 modifications critical for early embryonic gene regulation. These histone patterns are more broadly distributed in human oocytes than in mice [42].

Epigenetic reprogramming is highly sensitive to extrinsic perturbations. Assisted reproductive technologies (ART) and in vitro culture can alter methylation at imprinted loci, increasing the risk of disorders such as Beckwith–Wiedemann syndrome [17, 18]. Advanced maternal age exacerbates this instability, leading to global hypomethylation and histone deacetylase-mediated loss of acetylation in ovarian tissue, impairing oocyte quality [43]. High-resolution single-cell epigenomic mapping has revealed unexpected developmental plasticity in human embryos, offering insights into potential therapeutic targets [44].

In conclusion, epigenetic reprogramming in human germ cell development and preimplantation embryogenesis maintains a dynamic balance between the erasure and re-establishment of molecular signatures to ensure developmental integrity. High-resolution analysis has revealed both conserved and species-specific features, providing valuable information for translational applications in reproductive medicine.

3. Impact of cryopreservation on epigenetic stability

The intricate epigenetic reprogramming during gametogenesis and early embryogenesis establishes critical windows during which external stressors, such as those encountered during cryopreservation, may disrupt molecular fidelity. These dynamic phases of DNA demethylation and histone remodeling in primordial germ cells (PGCs) and early embryos heighten susceptibility to freezing stress, potentially leading to altered gene expression and developmental outcomes. Cryopreservation—encompassing slow freezing and vitrification—is a cornerstone of assisted reproduction, ensuring high survival, fertilization, cleavage, and embryo development rates. However, its potential to alter the epigenetic landscape of gametes and embryos raises concerns about long-term offspring safety. This section examines how cryopreservation affects epigenetic mechanisms.

3.1 DNA methylation alterations

Vitrification–warming can reduce DNA methylation levels at gene promoters, potentially leading to transcriptional dysregulation [45]. Evidence from bovine models indicates hypomethylation in essential developmental genes following vitrification [46]; however, these findings may not directly translate to humans due to species-specific differences in epigenetic regulation and reprogramming dynamics. For example, bovine embryos exhibit distinct methylation responses to cryopreservation, and methodological variability in human studies further limits the generalizability of conclusions [45]. Emerging technologies such as single-cell whole-genome bisulfite sequencing (scWGBS) now enable base-resolution methylome profiling, which may help reconcile these discrepancies. While global DNA methylation levels are generally maintained after cryopreservation, deviations can occur under suboptimal conditions [47]. Factors such as cryopreservation protocols, semen quality, and pre-existing epigenetic defects during spermatogenesis warrant further investigation [48]. Moreover, oxidative stress generated during cryopreservation—particularly in morphologically abnormal sperm—may indirectly disrupt epigenetic regulators, resulting in locus-specific hypo- or hypermethylation [49]. To ensure the safety of assisted reproductive technologies, future research should prioritize single-cell epigenomic analyses using human samples or non-human primate models to validate these findings.

3.2 Histone modifications

Histone post-translational modifications (PTMs) are critical for chromatin organization and gene regulation and are susceptible to cryopreservation-induced changes. Studies in bovine, porcine, and murine oocytes show that vitrification alters histone acetylation and methylation [50–52]. For instance, vitrification of oocytes is associated with decreased H3K9me3 and increased H3K9ac in cleavage-stage embryos, as well as reduced acetylation in blastocyst trophectoderm. Increased H4 acetylation and H3K9 methylation have also been reported in porcine and murine oocytes post-vitrification (**Table 1**) [53]. Current research focuses on H3 and H4, with limited data on H2A and H2B. Single-cell epigenomic approaches are expected to provide deeper insights [45].

3.3 Non-coding RNAs (ncRNAs)

Non-coding RNAs (ncRNAs)—including long ncRNAs (lncRNAs), microRNAs (miRNAs), small interfering RNAs (siRNAs), PIWI-interacting RNAs (piRNAs), and circular RNAs (circRNAs)—regulate transcription, pluripotency, meiosis, and early embryonic development [53–55]. miRNAs modulate gene expression via mRNA 3′UTR targeting, and their dysregulation in oocytes or embryos can lead to infertility and developmental anomalies [56]. Dicer, essential for siRNA biogenesis, is required for oocyte meiosis, and its loss causes meiotic arrest and chromosomal defects [56].

Vitrification–warming alters ncRNA profiles due to their environmental sensitivity. In mouse oocytes, 22 miRNAs were differentially expressed post-vitrification, including upregulation of miR-134-5p, miR-210-5p, and miR-21-3p, and downregulation of miR-465c-5p, targeting key metabolic genes (**Table 1**) [57]. PTEN expression, a negative regulator of the PI3K/AKT pathway critical for DNA repair and follicle activation, was reduced at transcript and protein levels [58]. Human RNA-seq studies show significant downregulation of lncRNAs in vitrified oocytes [59], though their roles in early embryogenesis remain unclear.

Molecular Endpoint	Human Findings	Bovine Findings	Mouse Findings
DNA Methylation	Global levels are generally stable post-vitrification; locus-specific changes in small studies	Hypomethylation in developmental genes	Partial demethylation at imprinted regions; ROS-induced hypo/hypermethylation
Histone Marks	Decreased H3K9me3 and increased H3K9ac in cleavage-stage embryos	Increased H4 acetylation and H3K9 methylation	Increased H4 acetylation and H3K9 methylation
Non-Coding RNAs	Significant downregulation of lncRNAs in vitrified oocytes	Limited data; suspected miRNA dysregulation	Altered miRNA expression
mtDNA Mutations	Oxidative damage leading to deletions; small heterogeneous studies	Higher mutation rate in cryopreserved embryos	Point mutations and impaired function due to cryostress

Table 1.
Comparison of molecular endpoints in human, bovine, and mouse models following cryopreservation.

The epigenetic consequences of cryopreservation vary by species and technical parameters, such as cryoprotectant type, cooling/warming rates, and freezing stage. In bovine models, cryopreserved oocytes exhibit reduced H3K9 acetylation, potentially affecting chromatin decondensation post-fertilization (**Table 1**) [60]. Blastocyst-stage cryopreservation can disrupt global DNA methylation and histone patterns, correlating with altered placental gene expression [61]. In ovarian tissue cryopreservation, ischemia–reperfusion injury during transplantation may alter follicular epigenomes [62]. For detailed impacts on genomic integrity, including DNA damage mechanisms, see Section 5.

In summary, while cryopreservation ensures high survival and developmental competence, accumulating evidence indicates it can affect epigenetic integrity via DNA methylation changes, histone PTM alterations, and ncRNA dysregulation. The clinical significance of these changes remains to be clarified. Integrating advanced single-cell epigenomic technologies with well-controlled, species-specific studies will be essential for ensuring the long-term safety of cryopreservation in reproductive medicine.

4. Human genome, genetic diseases, and genomic technologies

DNA is inherently vulnerable to chemical and physical insults under physiological conditions, leading to sequence alterations such as transpositions and base substitutions. These changes may result from replication, recombination, or repair errors, as well as from the intrinsic instability of nucleotide bonds at physiological temperature and pH [11, 63, 64]. In eukaryotic cells, genomic stability is maintained through the chromatin structure, in which DNA is packaged with histone and non-histone proteins to regulate accessibility and preserve gene function [65].

The mitochondrial genome (mtDNA), a 16.5 kb circular double-stranded molecule encoding 13 proteins, 22 tRNAs, and 2 rRNAs, is particularly prone to damage. Lacking histone protection and residing adjacent to the electron transport chain, mtDNA is highly susceptible to oxidative stress, resulting in a mutation rate roughly tenfold higher than that of nuclear DNA [66]. Damage to mtDNA can impair energy metabolism, directly affecting gamete viability and embryonic development.

According to the Online Mendelian Inheritance in Man (OMIM) database, genetic disorders such as cystic fibrosis, thalassemia, fragile X syndrome, and chromosomal abnormalities (e.g., trisomy 21 and trisomy 18) are strongly associated with infertility and embryonic developmental defects. These conditions may be exacerbated by environmental or physiological stressors that compromise genomic stability [12]. For individuals at elevated genetic risk, effective reproductive strategies require stringent genomic quality control to ensure optimal outcomes.

Advances in genomic technologies have transformed reproductive medicine. Next-generation sequencing (NGS) enables high-throughput detection of single-nucleotide variants, copy number alterations, and structural rearrangements across both nuclear and mitochondrial genomes. Single-cell sequencing provides insights into genomic heterogeneity, while long-read platforms, such as third-generation sequencing, enhance the resolution of complex genomic regions and structural variants [44]. Together, these technologies support comprehensive genomic assessment for fertility preservation and embryo evaluation.

5. Effects of cryopreservation on genomic integrity

Cryopreservation introduces physical and molecular stressors that may compromise genomic integrity in oocytes, sperm, and embryos, leading to chromosomal abnormalities, DNA fragmentation, and mutations. This section details these mechanisms.

5.1 Oocytes

Oocytes are particularly vulnerable to cryoinjury due to their large size (~100 μm in humans), high lipid content, and dynamic meiotic processes, which distinguish them from smaller somatic cells (10–20 μm) [67]. During spindle-sensitive meiotic stages, cryopreservation can disrupt microtubule assembly, resulting in chromosome misalignment and an increased risk of aneuploidy [68]. Animal studies, especially in mice, have reported elevated sister chromatid exchange (SCE)—a marker of mutagenesis—and DNA damage following cryopreservation [69]. Common cryoprotectants such as dimethyl sulfoxide (DMSO), propylene glycol, and ethylene glycol may exacerbate genomic stress by inducing DNA fragmentation, altering DNA methylation, or modifying gene expression profiles (**Table 2**) [70]. In addition, reactive oxygen species (ROS) generated during freezing contribute to spindle disassembly and DNA strand breaks, which can be detected using assays such as TUNEL and COMET (**Figure 2**) [71]. Although human studies using fluorescence in situ hybridization (FISH) or comprehensive chromosome screening have not demonstrated a consistent increase in chromosomal abnormalities [72], these investigations are limited by small sample sizes and incomplete chromosomal analyses. Moreover, while murine studies suggest that cryopreservation may increase SCE and DNA damage, such findings may not be fully applicable to humans due to species-specific differences, including oocyte size, lipid content, and meiotic dynamics. Human studies are further constrained by limited sample numbers and the absence of long-term follow-up, restricting our understanding of the sustained genomic impact of cryopreservation.

Vitrification has significantly improved oocyte survival rates (up to 96.9%) and pregnancy rates (65.2% per embryo transfer) compared to slow freezing, which historically yielded only a 2.3% pregnancy rate per thawed oocyte [73]. Despite these advances, clinical variability—stemming from differences in protocols, cryoprotectant exposure times, and embryologist expertise—may amplify genomic risks. For

Cryoprotectant	Typical Concentration	Reported Epigenetic/Genomic Effects
Dimethyl Sulfoxide (DMSO)	1.5–2 M	Induces DNA fragmentation; alters histone acetylation in oocytes
Propylene Glycol	1.5 M	Elevates intracellular calcium, leading to chromatin changes and hypermethylation at imprinted loci
Ethylene Glycol	1.5–2 M	Causes ROS-mediated mtDNA mutations; hypomethylation in developmental genes
Glycerol	1–2 M	Affects histone-modifying enzymes, resulting in altered methylation patterns

Table 2.
Summary of cryoprotectants, concentrations, and reported epigenetic/genomic effects.

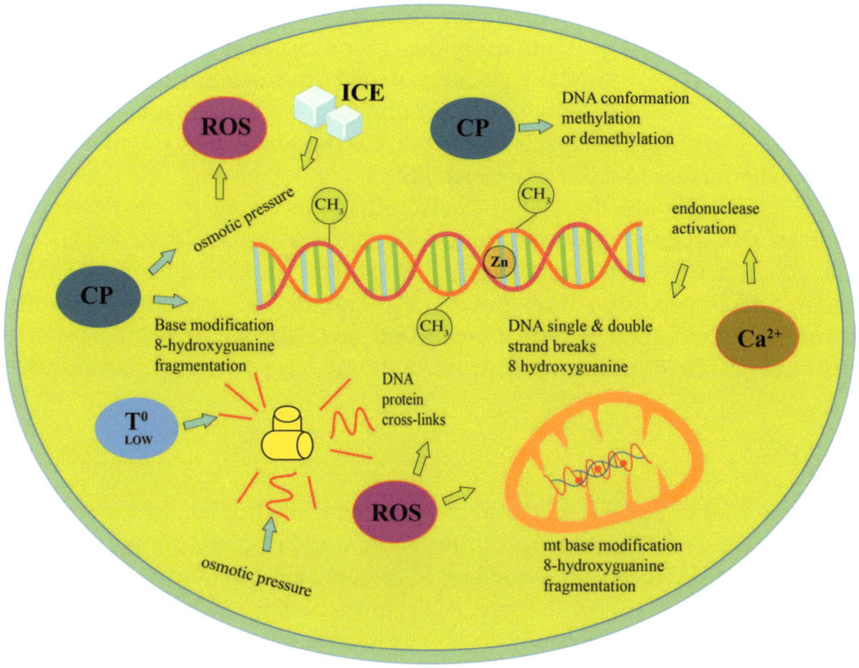

Figure 2.
The possible biological mechanisms of the effect of cryopreservation on the genome. ROS, reactive oxygen species; CP, cryoprotectants; T^0 *low, low temperature;* Ca^{2+}*, calcium; Zn, zinc molecule incorporated in DNA–protamine complex;* CH_3*, methylated DNA; ICE, a schematic representation of intracellular crystallization; yellow cylinders with red lines, schematic representation of centrosome with microtubules.*

instance, prolonged equilibration in propylene glycol increases genotoxicity by elevating intracellular calcium and altering chromatin structure (**Table 2**) [74]. Mouse studies demonstrate that optimized vitrification protocols, such as droplet systems or precise cryoloop handling, can reduce DNA fragmentation [75]. However, human data on SCE and COMET assay-based DNA damage are scarce, and no studies have explored cryoprotectant genotoxicity in human oocytes.

The long-term genomic safety of oocyte cryopreservation remains understudied. Retrospective data on over 900 babies born from cryopreserved oocytes report a low congenital anomaly rate (1.3%), but these studies lack standardized assessments and long-term follow-up [76]. The absence of prospective registries, such as the HOPE registry, limits our understanding of subtle epigenetic or mitochondrial DNA changes in offspring [77]. Clinical implications include the need for standardized protocols to minimize cryoinjury and informed consent addressing potential genomic risks. Future research should prioritize large-scale human studies on SCE, DNA fragmentation (via COMET assay), and cryoprotectant effects, alongside longitudinal offspring health studies to ensure the safety of vitrified oocytes, which are increasingly reported as comparable to fresh oocytes [78].

5.2 Sperm

Sperm cryopreservation, vital for assisted reproductive technologies, compromises genomic integrity through oxidative stress, osmotic injury, and chromatin decondensation. DNA fragmentation post-thaw varies significantly due to differences in cryopreservation techniques and individual cryoresistance, with sperm from infertile men showing greater damage due to reduced antioxidant defenses [79, 80]. Freezing may induce apoptosis or activate endonucleases, exacerbating DNA damage [81]. While fertilization capacity often persists, elevated DNA fragmentation is associated with increased miscarriage risk [82].

Antioxidants in cryomedia, such as melatonin or zinc, show partial protection against DNA damage in animal studies, but human data are limited [83]. Cryopreservation may also disrupt paternal epigenetic marks and telomere integrity, potentially affecting embryo development [84]. Long-term impacts on offspring remain understudied, though animal models suggest risks like aberrant growth [85]. Further research into optimized cryoprotectants and long-term outcomes is essential.

5.3 Embryos

Embryo cryopreservation, a critical component of in vitro fertilization (IVF), introduces stressors that may compromise genomic and epigenetic integrity, particularly during early cleavage stages when rapid cell division and chromatin remodeling heighten vulnerability to DNA damage. Both slow freezing and vitrification increase DNA fragmentation and potentially disrupt chromosomal stability, though vitrification is generally less damaging [86]. Cryoprotectants, such as ethylene glycol and 1,2-propanediol, can induce genomic stress independently of freezing, contributing to DNA fragmentation in animal models (**Figure 2**) [87]. While embryonic repair mechanisms may mitigate some damage during culture, the extent of protection remains unclear, necessitating further research into optimized protocols [88].

Although large studies report no significant increase in congenital anomalies, subtle epigenetic shifts, such as higher birth weights in babies from vitrified embryos, raise concerns about long-term effects [89]. Large-scale, prospective studies and standardized cryopreservation protocols are essential to fully evaluate the genomic and epigenetic safety of this vital reproductive technology.

5.4 Mitochondrial DNA

Cryopreservation significantly impacts the mitochondrial genome integrity in reproductive cells, leading to mtDNA mutations and functional impairments in sperm, oocytes, and gonadal tissue. In sperm, the lack of efficient mtDNA repair mechanisms results in increased mutation accumulation during cryopreservation, reducing semen quality, though intracytoplasmic sperm injection (ICSI) outcomes remain largely unaffected [90–93]. Oocyte cryopreservation, particularly vitrification, can disrupt mitochondrial functional gene expression and lower membrane potential ($\Delta\Psi m$), while inducing calcium imbalances that impair developmental competence (**Figure 2**) [94–96]. In gonadal tissue, the choice of cryoprotectant (e.g., DMSO outperforms glycerol and propanediol) is critical for preserving mitochondrial morphology and integrity [97]. Optimizing cryoprotectants and supplementing antioxidants like melatonin or glutathione ethyl ester can mitigate these damages [98–100]. Mitochondrial genomic integrity is particularly vulnerable. MtDNA lacks histones and has limited repair, making it prone to deletions and point mutations during cryopreservation. In cryopreserved oocytes, mtDNA copy number decreases, impairing energy production and embryo development (**Table 1**) [101]. Research shows that resveratrol promotes mitochondrial recovery from cryopreservation-induced damage in oocytes and embryos [102]. Studies show that supplementing oocytes with extra mtDNA can restore function, but transmission efficiency varies [103]. Transgenerational effects are evident, with altered mtDNA in offspring potentially linked to metabolic issues [104]. Integrating nuclear and mitochondrial assessments is vital for comprehensive genomic evaluation in fertility preservation.

6. Advances in genetic and reproductive technologies for fertility preservation

6.1 Female fertility preservation technologies

Recent advances in female fertility preservation have significantly improved options for women facing fertility-threatening conditions such as cancer treatments or premature ovarian insufficiency. Oocyte cryopreservation via vitrification is now the gold standard for post-pubertal women, with live birth rates reaching ~32% [105]. This method avoids ethical concerns associated with embryo freezing (which requires sperm and has a higher success rate of ~41%) but is less suitable for prepubertal girls [105, 106]. For these younger patients, ovarian tissue cryopreservation (OTC) remains the only option, allowing restoration of both fertility and endocrine function upon transplantation, with reported live birth rates of 21% (IVF) and 33% (natural conception). Emerging techniques like in vitro maturation (IVM) of immature oocytes combined with vitrification offer a hormone-free alternative for hormone-sensitive cancers, though success rates remain low due to suboptimal culture conditions [106]. Additionally, artificial ovary bioengineering and follicle encapsulation are experimental approaches aiming to improve graft survival and reduce ischemic damage. Future directions include AI-assisted follicle monitoring and automated vitrification protocols to enhance efficiency [107].

6.2 Male fertility preservation technologies

For males, sperm cryopreservation remains the most established method, with post-thaw fertilization rates of 60–93%. However, cryodamage from oxidative stress remains a challenge; antioxidants like melatonin have shown promise in improving sperm motility and DNA integrity [108]. For prepubertal boys who lack mature sperm, testicular tissue cryopreservation and spermatogonial stem cell (SSC) banking are experimental but promising. SSCs can be cryopreserved and later transplanted or differentiated in vitro to produce functional sperm. Melatonin supplementation enhances SSC survival and proliferation, mitigating chemotherapy-induced damage. Xenografting (transplanting human testicular tissue into immunodeficient mice) has demonstrated sperm production in animal models, though ethical and safety concerns limit clinical translation [108]. Emerging gene-editing techniques (e.g., CRISPR) may further optimize SSC culture and differentiation, while microfluidic sperm sorting and AI-based sperm selection could improve assisted reproductive outcomes [107].

These advances highlight the rapid progress in fertility preservation, though standardization of experimental techniques and ethical considerations remain critical for broader clinical adoption. Additionally, recent technological strides have enhanced our ability to probe and improve epigenetic and genomic outcomes in fertility preservation. Next-generation sequencing (NGS) enables detailed epigenomic profiling, revealing cryopreservation-induced changes in methylation landscapes [61]. Single-cell RNA-seq and ATAC-seq provide insights into chromatin accessibility in preserved gametes [109]. In reproductive technologies, mitochondrial replacement therapies (MRT) like pronuclear transfer mitigate mtDNA defects [110]. Preimplantation genetic testing (PGT) screens for aneuploidy and mutations, improving the selection of viable embryos post-cryopreservation [111]. Epigenetic clocks, based on methylation patterns, assess biological aging in gametes, predicting fertility outcomes [112]. Advances in cryoprotectants, such as nanoparticle-based agents, reduce toxicity and preserve integrity [113]. These innovations bridge genetics and epigenetics, fostering safer fertility preservation.

Importantly, CRISPR-based epigenetic editing offers a promising strategy to mitigate cryopreservation-induced epigenetic abnormalities [114]. For example, CRISPR/Cas9-dCas9 systems can precisely modulate DNA methylation or histone modifications at specific loci, such as imprinting control regions, potentially correcting hypomethylation or aberrant chromatin states caused by cryostorage. In animal models, CRISPR has been successfully applied to restore developmental epigenetic marks essential for embryogenesis [115]. However, major challenges remain before clinical translation, including risks of off-target genomic alterations and the unknown intergenerational consequences of germline epigenetic editing. Furthermore, stringent global regulatory frameworks (e.g., FDA and EMA) and ethical debates surrounding germline modification necessitate thorough safety validation before clinical use. Future research should prioritize non-human primate models and integrative multi-omics approaches to evaluate the long-term safety and efficacy of CRISPR-based epigenetic interventions in fertility preservation.

7. Strategies to preserve epigenetic fidelity and minimize genomic damage

Mitigating epigenetic and genomic risks in fertility preservation requires a dual approach combining biochemical interventions and technical optimization. Key antioxidants demonstrate multi-level protection: Resveratrol significantly reduces ROS-induced DNA damage [61], while zinc plays a pivotal role in maintaining epigenetic stability. Post-chemotherapy Zn supplementation restored normal DNA methylation patterns, preserved spermatogonial stem cells, and reduced sperm DNA fragmentation by >50% ($P < 0.001$) (**Figure 2**). These effects are enhanced when combined with optimized vitrification protocols employing controlled cooling rates to prevent ice crystal-induced chromatin damage [45]. Post-thaw recovery benefits from HDAC inhibitors like valproic acid for histone modification repair [116], alongside novel mitochondrial interventions such as autologous mitochondrial transfer to safely restore mtDNA copy number [117].

The strategy hierarchy should prioritize: (1) Pre-preservation preparation through dietary micronutrients (folate/B-vitamins) and exercise to establish epigenetic resilience; (2) Cryopreservation with antioxidant-fortified media and precision cooling protocols; (3) Post-thaw epigenetic rehabilitation using targeted modulators. Current evidence underscores zinc's unique dual functionality in both epigenetic maintenance (DNMT support) and structural chromatin protection [61, 118], warranting its inclusion in standard protocols. Longitudinal studies are needed to establish optimal antioxidant dosing thresholds and validate the safety of epigenetic modulator cocktails [119].

8. Challenges, ethical considerations, and future directions

Fertility preservation techniques, such as cryopreservation and in vitro maturation, face persistent challenges in maintaining the integrity of epigenetic and genomic information. Cryopreservation may trigger abnormal epigenetic changes, such as DNA methylation, in imprinted regions, posing potential threats to embryonic development and offspring health [120]. Similarly, in vitro culture can also cause oxidative stress, potentially leading to DNA damage and chromosomal abnormalities. Factors such as individual sperm or egg quality differences and the sensitivity of cryopreservation agents further increase the complexity of the results, and currently, there is a lack of long-term data support for potential intergenerational effects and ethical issues, such as emerging technologies like gene editing [121].

Ethical considerations involve not only the effectiveness of the technology but also aspects such as informed consent, regulatory oversight, and public participation. For example, the US Food and Drug Administration (FDA) classifies mitochondrial replacement therapy (MRT) as an experimental therapy due to potential genetic risks, while the European Medicines Agency (EMA) allows its use under strict conditions in specific regions [122, 123]. MRT policies vary greatly around the world - some countries regulate MRT along with gene editing technologies, while others (such as the United Kingdom through the HFEA) adopt specific and detailed regulatory frameworks. Many countries are beginning to involve the public in policy discussions on MRT, but few have established mechanisms for participatory democracy in the field of reproductive technology. Informed consent for fertility preservation should clearly state the potential epigenetic risks, such as: "Cryopreservation may lead to subtle molecular changes in reproductive cells or embryos, including DNA methylation or changes in mitochondrial function, which may have unknown long-term effects on offspring health. Suggest continuous monitoring".

To address these challenges, long-term monitoring through multi-center registration systems is crucial for tracking the epigenetic and genomic markers of offspring from assisted reproductive technologies. Advanced tools, such as whole-genome bisulfite sequencing, single-cell sequencing, and non-human primate models, will be essential for detecting subtle molecular abnormalities and elucidating intergenerational effects [120]. Standardizing cryopreservation protocols across centers will further reduce differences and enhance data reliability.

Looking to the future, future strategies should focus on optimizing cryopreservation agents, exploring innovative preservation methods such as freeze-drying or nano-heating, and leveraging multi-omics data integration with artificial intelligence-based predictive models. Epigenetic editing based on CRISPR is expected to correct changes caused by cryopreservation, while stem cell-derived gametes and artificial reproductive tissues may provide alternative approaches for fertility preservation [121]. Ultimately, interdisciplinary collaboration among reproductive biologists, bioengineers, clinicians, ethicists, and policymakers will be crucial for establishing safe, effective, and ethical fertility preservation practices and minimizing risks to epigenetic and genomic integrity.

9. Conclusions

Fertility preservation techniques, while transformative, pose risks to epigenetic stability and genomic integrity through mechanisms like altered DNA methylation, histone modifications, and mitochondrial damage. Advances in genetic and reproductive technologies offer tools to mitigate these effects, with strategies emphasizing protective agents, refined protocols, and monitoring. By prioritizing epigenetic fidelity, we can enhance the safety and efficacy of these practices, safeguarding transgenerational health. Continued research is imperative to standardize approaches and address emerging challenges, ultimately empowering individuals in their reproductive journeys.

Acknowledgements

This work was supported by grants from the Research Program for Medicine and Health of Zhejiang Province [2021KY080 (L.Y.) and 2025KY581 (C.W.)] and the "Pioneer" and "Leading Goose" R&D Program of Zhejiang [2024C03004 (X.T.)].

Conflict of interest

The authors declare no conflict of interest.

Author details

Songlin Zhang[1], Chenglu Wang[2], Leixiang Yang[1], Min Zheng[2], Xiaohua Tang[1*] and Xiaopan Chen[1*]

1 Laboratory Medicine Center, Department of Genetic and Genomic Medicine, Zhejiang Provincial People's Hospital (Affiliated People's Hospital), Hangzhou Medical College, Hangzhou, Zhejiang, China

2 Center for Reproductive Medicine, Department of Reproductive Endocrinology, Zhejiang Provincial People's Hospital (Affiliated People's Hospital), Hangzhou Medical College, Hangzhou, Zhejiang, China

*Address all correspondence to: tsh006@126.com
and chenxiaopan@hmc.edu.cn

References

[1] Donnez J, Dolmans MM. Fertility preservation in women. Campion EW, editor. The New England Journal of Medicine. 2017;**377**(17):1657-1665

[2] Donnez J, Dolmans MM. Fertility preservation in men and women: Where are we in 2021? Are we rising to the challenge? Fertility and Sterility. 2021;**115**(5):1089-1090

[3] Cascante SD, Berkeley AS, Licciardi F, McCaffrey C, Grifo JA. Planned oocyte cryopreservation: The state of the ART. Reproductive Biomedicine Online. 2023;**47**(6):103367

[4] Vinolas C, Raad J, Sonigo C, Sifer C, Sermondade N, Grynberg M. Medical techniques of fertility preservation in the male and female. Journal of Visceral Surgery. 2018;**155**:S3-S9

[5] Shorokhova M, Pugovkina N, Zemelko V, Lyublinskaya O, Grinchuk T. Long-term cryopreservation may cause genomic instability and the premature senescence of cells. International Journal of Molecular Sciences. 2024;**25**(3):1467

[6] Sindik N, Pereza N, Dević PS. Epigenetics of oogenesis. Archives of Gynecology and Obstetrics. 2025;**311**(2):183-190

[7] Ben Maamar M, Nilsson EE, Skinner MK. Epigenetic transgenerational inheritance, gametogenesis and germline development†. Biology of Reproduction. 2021;**105**(3):570-592

[8] Tang WWC, Kobayashi T, Irie N, Dietmann S, Surani MA. Specification and epigenetic programming of the human germ line. Nature Reviews Genetics. 2016;**17**(10):585-600

[9] Shirane K, Lorincz M. Epigenetic mechanisms governing female and male germline development in mammals. Sexual Development. 2022;**16**(5-6):365-387

[10] Singh A, Rappolee DA, Ruden DM. Epigenetic reprogramming in mice and humans: From fertilization to primordial germ cell development. Cells. 2023;**12**(14):1874

[11] Lindahl T. Instability and decay of the primary structure of DNA. Nature. 1993;**362**(6422):709-715

[12] McCarthy MJ, Baumber J, Kass PH, Meyers SA. Osmotic stress induces oxidative cell damage to rhesus macaque spermatozoa. Biology of Reproduction. 2010;**82**(3):644-651

[13] Kültz D, Chakravarty D. Maintenance of genomic integrity in mammalian kidney cells exposed to hyperosmotic stress. Comparative Biochemistry and Physiology Part A: Molecular & Integrative Physiology. 2001;**130**(3):421-428

[14] Gualtieri R, Kalthur G, Barbato V, Di Nardo M, Adiga SK, Talevi R. Mitochondrial dysfunction and oxidative stress caused by cryopreservation in reproductive cells. Antioxidants. 2021;**10**(3):337

[15] Lee MT, Bonneau AR, Giraldez AJ. Zygotic genome activation during the maternal-to-zygotic transition. Annual Review of Cell and Developmental Biology. 2014;**30**:581-613

[16] Burton A, Torres-Padilla ME. Chromatin dynamics in the regulation of cell fate allocation during early embryogenesis. Nature

Reviews Molecular Cell Biology. 2014;**15**(11):723-734

[17] Greenberg MVC, Bourc'his D. The diverse roles of DNA methylation in mammalian development and disease. Nature Reviews Molecular Cell Biology. 2019;**20**(10):590-607

[18] Jambhekar A, Dhall A, Shi Y. Roles and regulation of histone methylation in animal development. Nature Reviews Molecular Cell Biology. 2019;**20**(10):625-641

[19] Surani MA, Hayashi K, Hajkova P. Genetic and epigenetic regulators of pluripotency. Cell. 2007;**128**(4):747-762

[20] Ohinata Y, Ohta H, Shigeta M, Yamanaka K, Wakayama T, Saitou M. A signaling principle for the specification of the germ cell lineage in mice. Cell. 2009;**137**(3):571-584

[21] Bao S, Tang F, Li X, Hayashi K, Gillich A, Lao K, et al. Epigenetic reversion of post-implantation epiblast to pluripotent embryonic stem cells. Nature. 2009;**461**(7268):1292-1295

[22] Seki Y, Hayashi K, Itoh K, Mizugaki M, Saitou M, Matsui Y. Extensive and orderly reprogramming of genome-wide chromatin modifications associated with specification and early development of germ cells in mice. Developmental Biology. 2005;**278**(2):440-458

[23] Seki Y, Yamaji M, Yabuta Y, Sano M, Shigeta M, Matsui Y, et al. Cellular dynamics associated with the genome-wide epigenetic reprogramming in migrating primordial germ cells in mice. Development (Cambridge England). 2007;**134**(14):2627-2638

[24] Hajkova P, Ancelin K, Waldmann T, Lacoste N, Lange UC, Cesari F, et al. Chromatin dynamics during epigenetic reprogramming in the mouse germ line. Nature. 2008;**452**(7189):877-881

[25] Sasaki H, Matsui Y. Epigenetic events in mammalian germ-cell development: Reprogramming and beyond. Nature Reviews Genetics. 2008;**9**(2):129-140

[26] de Sousa C, Lopes SM, Hayashi K, Shovlin TC, Mifsud W, Surani MA, et al. X chromosome activity in mouse XX primordial germ cells. PLoS Genetics. 2008;**4**(2):e30

[27] Matsui Y, Zsebo K, Hogan BL. Derivation of pluripotential embryonic stem cells from murine primordial germ cells in culture. Cell. 1992;**70**(5):841-847

[28] Tada T, Tada M, Hilton K, Barton SC, Sado T, Takagi N, et al. Epigenotype switching of imprintable loci in embryonic germ cells. Development Genes and Evolution. 1998;**207**(8):551-561

[29] Ancelin K, Lange UC, Hajkova P, Schneider R, Bannister AJ, Kouzarides T, et al. Blimp1 associates with Prmt5 and directs histone arginine methylation in mouse germ cells. Nature Cell Biology. 2006;**8**(6):623-630

[30] Tee WW, Pardo M, Theunissen TW, Yu L, Choudhary JS, Hajkova P, et al. Prmt5 is essential for early mouse development and acts in the cytoplasm to maintain ES cell pluripotency. Genes & Development. 2010;**24**(24):2772-2777

[31] Bostick M, Kim JK, Estève PO, Clark A, Pradhan S, Jacobsen SE. UHRF1 plays a role in maintaining DNA methylation in mammalian cells. Science. 2007;**317**(5845):1760-1764

[32] Tachibana M, Matsumura Y, Fukuda M, Kimura H, Shinkai Y. G9a/GLP complexes independently mediate

H3K9 and DNA methylation to silence transcription. The EMBO Journal. 2008;**27**(20):2681-2690

[33] Hajkova P, Erhardt S, Lane N, Haaf T, El-Maarri O, Reik W, et al. Epigenetic reprogramming in mouse primordial germ cells. Mechanisms of Development. 2002;**117**(1-2):15-23

[34] West JA, Viswanathan SR, Yabuuchi A, Cunniff K, Takeuchi A, Park IH, et al. A role for Lin28 in primordial germ-cell development and germ-cell malignancy. Nature. 2009;**460**(7257):909-913

[35] Pichler G, Wolf P, Schmidt CS, Meilinger D, Schneider K, Frauer C, et al. Cooperative DNA and histone binding by Uhrf2 links the two major repressive epigenetic pathways. Journal of Cellular Biochemistry. 2011;**112**(9):2585-2593

[36] Popp C, Dean W, Feng S, Cokus SJ, Andrews S, Pellegrini M, et al. Genome-wide erasure of DNA methylation in mouse primordial germ cells is affected by AID deficiency. Nature. 2010;**463**(7284):1101-1105

[37] Lane N, Dean W, Erhardt S, Hajkova P, Surani A, Walter J, et al. Resistance of IAPs to methylation reprogramming may provide a mechanism for epigenetic inheritance in the mouse. Genesis. 2003;**35**(2):88-93

[38] Maatouk DM, Kellam LD, Mann MRW, Lei H, Li E, Bartolomei MS, et al. DNA methylation is a primary mechanism for silencing postmigratory primordial germ cell genes in both germ cell and somatic cell lineages. Development (Cambridge England). 2006;**133**(17):3411-3418

[39] Gu TP, Guo F, Yang H, Wu HP, Xu GF, Liu W, et al. The role of Tet3 DNA dioxygenase in epigenetic reprogramming by oocytes. Nature. 2011;**477**(7366):606-610

[40] Hackett JA, Zylicz JJ, Surani MA. Parallel mechanisms of epigenetic reprogramming in the germline. Trends in Genetics. 2012;**28**(4):164-174

[41] Dahl JA, Jung I, Aanes H, Greggains GD, Manaf A, Lerdrup M, et al. Broad histone H3K4me3 domains in mouse oocytes modulate maternal-to-zygotic transition. Nature. 2016;**537**(7621):548-552

[42] Zhang B, Zheng H, Huang B, Li W, Xiang Y, Peng X, et al. Allelic reprogramming of the histone modification H3K4me3 in early mammalian development. Nature. 2016;**537**(7621):553-557

[43] Voros C, Varthaliti A, Mavrogianni D, Athanasiou D, Athanasiou A, Athanasiou A, et al. Epigenetic alterations in ovarian function and their impact on assisted reproductive technologies: A systematic review. Biomedicine. 2025;**13**(3):730

[44] Wang Y, Yuan P, Yan Z, Yang M, Huo Y, Nie Y, et al. Single-cell multiomics sequencing reveals the functional regulatory landscape of early embryos. Nature Communications. 2021;**12**(1):1247

[45] Liu Y, Chen J, Chian RC. Beyond survival effects of vitrification-warming on epigenetic modification and maternal transcripts of oocytes. In: Embryology Update. London: IntechOpen; 2022

[46] Chen H, Zhang L, Deng T, Zou P, Wang Y, Quan F, et al. Effects of oocyte vitrification on epigenetic status in early bovine embryos. Theriogenology. 2016;**86**(3):868-878

[47] Depincé A, Gabory A, Dziewulska K, Le Bail P, Jammes H, Labbé C. DNA

methylation stability in fish spermatozoa upon external constraint: Impact of fish hormonal stimulation and sperm cryopreservation. Molecular Reproduction and Development. 2020;**87**(1):124-134

[48] Khosravizadeh Z, Hassanzadeh G, Tavakkoly Bazzaz J, Alizadeh F, Totonchi M, Salehi E, et al. The effect of cryopreservation on DNA methylation patterns of the chromosome 15q11–q13 region in human spermatozoa. Cell and Tissue Banking. 2020;**21**(3):433-445

[49] Guillaumet-Adkins A, Yañez Y, Peris-Diaz MD, Calabria I, Palanca-Ballester C, Sandoval J. Epigenetics and oxidative stress in aging. Oxidative Medicine and Cellular Longevity. 2017;**2017**(1):9175806

[50] Spinaci M, Vallorani C, Bucci D, Tamanini C, Porcu E, Galeati G. Vitrification of pig oocytes induces changes in histone H4 acetylation and histone H3 lysine 9 methylation (H3K9). Veterinary Research Communications. 2012;**36**(3):165-171

[51] Yan LY, Yan J, Qiao J, Zhao PL, Liu P. Effects of oocyte vitrification on histone modifications. Reproduction, Fertility, and Development. 2010;**22**(6):920-925

[52] Suo L, Meng Q, Pei Y, Fu X, Wang Y, Bunch TD, et al. Effect of cryopreservation on acetylation patterns of lysine 12 of histone H4 (acH4K12) in mouse oocytes and zygotes. Journal of Assisted Reproduction and Genetics. 2010;**27**(12):735-741

[53] Beermann J, Piccoli MT, Viereck J, Thum T. Non-coding RNAs in development and disease: Background, mechanisms, and therapeutic approaches. Physiological Reviews. 2016;**96**(4):1297-1325

[54] Suh N, Blelloch R. Small RNAs in early mammalian development: From gametes to gastrulation. Development (Cambridge England). 2011;**138**(9):1653-1661

[55] O'Brien J, Hayder H, Zayed Y, Peng C. Overview of MicroRNA biogenesis, mechanisms of actions, and circulation. Frontiers in Endocrinology. 2018;**9**:402

[56] Salas-Huetos A, James ER, Aston KI, Jenkins TG, Carrell DT, Yeste M. The expression of miRNAs in human ovaries, oocytes, extracellular vesicles, and early embryos: A systematic review. Cells. 2019;**8**(12):1564

[57] Li J, Yang X, Liu F, Song Y, Liu Y. Evaluation of differentially expressed microRNAs in vitrified oocytes by next generation sequencing. The International Journal of Biochemistry & Cell Biology. 2019;**112**:134-140

[58] Maidarti M, Anderson RA, Telfer EE. Crosstalk between PTEN/PI3K/akt signalling and DNA damage in the oocyte: Implications for primordial follicle activation, oocyte quality and ageing. Cells. 2020;**9**(1):200

[59] Huo Y, Yuan P, Qin Q, Yan Z, Yan L, Liu P, et al. Effects of vitrification and cryostorage duration on single-cell RNA-seq profiling of vitrified-thawed human metaphase II oocytes. Frontiers in Medicine. 2021;**15**(1):144-154

[60] Barberet J, Barry F, Choux C, Guilleman M, Karoui S, Simonot R. What impact does oocyte vitrification have on epigenetics and gene expression? Clinical Epigenetics. 2020;**12**(1):121

[61] Saftić Martinović L, Mladenić T, Lovrić D, Ostojić S, Dević Pavlić S. Decoding the epigenetics of infertility: Mechanisms, environmental influences,

and therapeutic strategies. Epigenomes. 2024;**8**(3):34

[62] Trapphoff T, Dieterle S. Cryopreservation of ovarian and testicular tissue and the influence on epigenetic pattern. International Journal of Molecular Sciences. 2023;**24**(13):11061

[63] Lindahl T, Karlström O. Heat-induced depyrimidination of deoxyribonucleic acid in neutral solution. Biochemistry. 1973;**12**(25):5151-5154

[64] Finnegan DJ. Transposable elements and DNA transposition in eukaryotes. Current Opinion in Cell Biology. 1990;**2**(3):471-477

[65] Ljungman M, Hanawalt PC. Efficient protection against oxidative DNA damage in chromatin. Molecular Carcinogenesis. 1992;**5**(4):264-269

[66] Yakes FM, Van Houten B. Mitochondrial DNA damage is more extensive and persists longer than nuclear DNA damage in human cells following oxidative stress. Proceedings of the National Academy of Sciences of the United States of America. 1997;**94**(2):514-519

[67] Zhou GB, Li N. Bovine oocytes cryoinjury and how to improve their development following cryopreservation. Animal Biotechnology. 2013;**24**(2):94-106

[68] Bromfield JJ, Coticchio G, Hutt K, Sciajno R, Borini A, Albertini DF. Meiotic spindle dynamics in human oocytes following slow-cooling cryopreservation. Human Reproduction (Oxford England). 2009;**24**(9):2114-2123

[69] Huang JYJ, Chen HY, Park JYS, Tan SL, Chian RC. Comparison of spindle and chromosome configuration in in vitro- and in vivo-matured mouse oocytes after vitrification. Fertility and Sterility. 2008;**90**(4 Suppl):1424-1432

[70] Bouquet M, Selva J, Auroux M. Cryopreservation of mouse oocytes: Mutagenic effects in the embryo? Biology of Reproduction. 1993;**49**(4):764-769

[71] Dizdaroglu M, Jaruga P. Mechanisms of free radical-induced damage to DNA. Free Radical Research. 2012;**46**(4):382-419

[72] Forman EJ, Li X, Ferry KM, Scott K, Treff NR, Scott RT. Oocyte vitrification does not increase the risk of embryonic aneuploidy or diminish the implantation potential of blastocysts created after intracytoplasmic sperm injection: A novel, paired randomized controlled trial using DNA fingerprinting. Fertility and Sterility. 2012;**98**(3):644-649

[73] Bolton VN, Hayden C, Robinson M, Abdo D, Pericleous-Smith A, Association of Reproductive and Clinical Scientists and British Fertility Society. Human oocyte cryopreservation: Revised evidence for practice. Human Fertility (Cambridge, England). 2023;**26**(1):2-16

[74] Berthelot-Ricou A, Perrin J, di Giorgio C, de Meo M, Botta A, Courbiere B. Assessment of 1,2-propanediol (PrOH) genotoxicity on mouse oocytes by comet assay. Fertility and Sterility. 2011;**96**(4):1002-1007

[75] Stachowiak EM, Papis K, Kruszewski M, Iwaneńko T, Bartłomiejczyk T, Modliński JA. Comparison of the level(s) of DNA damage using comet assay in bovine oocytes subjected to selected vitrification methods. Reproduction in Domestic Animals. 2009;**44**(4):653-658

[76] Noyes N, Porcu E, Borini A. Over 900 oocyte cryopreservation babies born with no apparent increase in congenital

anomalies. Reproductive Biomedicine Online. 2009;**18**(6):769-776

[77] Ezcurra D, Rangnow J, Craig M, Schertz J. The HOPE registry: First US registry for oocyte cryopreservation. Reproductive Biomedicine Online. 2008;**17**(6):743-744

[78] Cobo A, Meseguer M, Remohí J, Pellicer A. Use of cryo-banked oocytes in an ovum donation programme: A prospective, randomized, controlled, clinical trial. Human Reproduction (Oxford England). 2010;**25**(9):2239-2246

[79] Kalthur G, Adiga SK, Upadhya D, Rao S, Kumar P. Effect of cryopreservation on sperm DNA integrity in patients with teratospermia. Fertility and Sterility. 2008;**89**(6):1723-1727

[80] Zribi N, Chakroun NF, El Euch H, Gargouri J, Bahloul A, Keskes LA. Effects of cryopreservation on human sperm deoxyribonucleic acid integrity. Fertility and Sterility. 2010;**93**(1):159-166

[81] Thomson LK, Fleming SD, Barone K, Zieschang JA, Clark AM. The effect of repeated freezing and thawing on human sperm DNA fragmentation. Fertility and Sterility. 2010;**93**(4):1147-1156

[82] Robinson L, Gallos ID, Conner SJ, Rajkhowa M, Miller D, Lewis S, et al. The effect of sperm DNA fragmentation on miscarriage rates: A systematic review and meta-analysis. Human Reproduction (Oxford England). 2012;**27**(10):2908-2917

[83] Branco CS, Garcez ME, Pasqualotto FF, Erdtman B, Salvador M. Resveratrol and ascorbic acid prevent DNA damage induced by cryopreservation in human semen. Cryobiology. 2010;**60**(2):235-237

[84] Valcarce DG, Cartón-García F, Riesco MF, Herráez MP, Robles V. Analysis of DNA damage after human sperm cryopreservation in genes crucial for fertilization and early embryo development. Andrology. 2013;**1**(5):723-730

[85] Fernández-Gonzalez R, Moreira PN, Pérez-Crespo M, Sánchez-Martín M, Ramirez MA, Pericuesta E, et al. Long-term effects of mouse intracytoplasmic sperm injection with DNA-fragmented sperm on health and behavior of adult offspring. Biology of Reproduction. 2008;**78**(4):761-772

[86] Li L, Zhang X, Zhao L, Xia X, Wang W. Comparison of DNA apoptosis in mouse and human blastocysts after vitrification and slow freezing. Molecular Reproduction and Development. 2012;**79**(3):229-236

[87] Rajaei F, Karja NWK, Agung B, Wongsrikeao P, Taniguchi M, Murakami M, et al. Analysis of DNA fragmentation of porcine embryos exposed to cryoprotectants. Reproduction in Domestic Animals. 2005;**40**(5):429-432

[88] Kopeika J, Thornhill A, Khalaf Y. The effect of cryopreservation on the genome of gametes and embryos: Principles of cryobiology and critical appraisal of the evidence. Human Reproduction Update. 2015;**21**(2):209-227

[89] Levi Setti PE, Albani E, Morenghi E, Morreale G, Delle Piane L, Scaravelli G, et al. Comparative analysis of fetal and neonatal outcomes of pregnancies from fresh and cryopreserved/thawed oocytes in the same group of patients. Fertility and Sterility. 2013;**100**(2):396-401

[90] Zinovkin RA, Zamyatnin AA. Mitochondria-targeted drugs. Current Molecular Pharmacology. 2019;**12**(3):202-214

[91] Gualtieri R, Mollo V, Duma G, Talevi R. Redox control of surface protein sulphhydryls in bovine spermatozoa reversibly modulates sperm adhesion to the oviductal epithelium and capacitation. Reproduction (Cambridge England). 2009;**138**(1):33-43

[92] Clapham DE. Calcium signaling. Cell. 2007;**131**(6):1047-1058

[93] Rosati AJ, Whitcomb BW, Brandon N, Buck Louis GM, Mumford SL, Schisterman EF, et al. Sperm mitochondrial DNA biomarkers and couple fecundity. Human Reproduction (Oxford England). 2020;**35**(11):2619-2625

[94] Zhang F, Zhang ZY, Cai MD, Li XX, Li YH, Lei Y, et al. Effect of vitrification temperature and cryoprotectant concentrations on the mRNA transcriptome of bovine mature oocytes after vitrifying at immature stage. Theriogenology. 2020;**148**:225-235

[95] Chen C, Han S, Liu W, Wang Y, Huang G. Effect of vitrification on mitochondrial membrane potential in human metaphase II oocytes. Journal of Assisted Reproduction and Genetics. 2012;**29**(10):1045-1050

[96] Larman MG, Sheehan CB, Gardner DK. Calcium-free vitrification reduces cryoprotectant-induced zona pellucida hardening and increases fertilization rates in mouse oocytes. Reproduction (Cambridge England). 2006;**131**(1):53-61

[97] Mailloux RJ. An update on mitochondrial reactive oxygen species production. Antioxidants. 2020;**9**(6):472

[98] Ruihuan G, Zhichao L, Song G, Jing F, Yijuan S, Xiaoxi S. Oocyte vitrification temporarily turns on oxidation-reduction process genes in mouse preimplantation embryos. Reproductive Sciences (Thousand Oaks, California). 2021;**28**(5):1307-1315

[99] Eroglu B, Szurek EA, Schall P, Latham KE, Eroglu A. Probing lasting cryoinjuries to oocyte-embryo transcriptome. PLoS One. 2020;**15**(4):e0231108

[100] Tan DX, Manchester LC, Qin L, Reiter RJ. Melatonin: A mitochondrial targeting molecule involving mitochondrial protection and dynamics. International Journal of Molecular Sciences. 2016;**17**(12):2124

[101] Cagnone GLM, Tsai TS, Makanji Y, Matthews P, Gould J, Bonkowski MS, et al. Restoration of normal embryogenesis by mitochondrial supplementation in pig oocytes exhibiting mitochondrial DNA deficiency. Scientific Reports. 2016;**6**:23229

[102] Iwata H. Resveratrol enhanced mitochondrial recovery from cryopreservation-induced damages in oocytes and embryos. Reproductive Medicine and Biology. 2021;**20**(4):419-426

[103] St John JC, Andreas E, Penn A. Can the supplementation of oocytes with extra copies of mtDNA impact development without being transmitted? A molecular account. International Journal of Molecular Sciences. 2025;**26**(6):2746

[104] Jansen RPS, Burton GJ. Mitochondrial dysfunction in reproduction. Mitochondrion. 2004;**4**(5-6):577-600

[105] Fraison E, Huberlant S, Labrune E, Cavalieri M, Montagut M, Brugnon F, et al. Live birth rate after female fertility preservation for cancer or

haematopoietic stem cell transplantation: A systematic review and meta-analysis of the three main techniques; embryo, oocyte and ovarian tissue cryopreservation. Human Reproduction (Oxford England). 2023;**38**(3):489-502

[106] Son WY, Henderson S, Cohen Y, Dahan M, Buckett W. Immature oocyte for fertility preservation. Frontiers in Endocrinology. 2019;**10**:464

[107] Medenica S, Zivanovic D, Batkoska L, Marinelli S, Basile G, Perino A, et al. The future is coming: Artificial intelligence in the treatment of infertility could improve assisted reproduction outcomes-the value of regulatory frameworks. Diagnostics (Basel, Switzerland). 2022;**12**(12):2979

[108] Sun TC, Li HY, Li XY, Yu K, Deng SL, Tian L. Protective effects of melatonin on male fertility preservation and reproductive system. Cryobiology. 2020;**95**:1-8

[109] Wilkinson AL, Zorzan I, Rugg-Gunn PJ. Epigenetic regulation of early human embryo development. Cell Stem Cell. 2023;**30**(12):1569-1584

[110] Tachibana M, Kuno T, Yaegashi N. Mitochondrial replacement therapy and assisted reproductive technology: A paradigm shift toward treatment of genetic diseases in gametes or in early embryos. Reproductive Medicine and Biology. 2018;**17**(4):421-433

[111] Harper JC, Aittomäki K, Borry P, Cornel MC, de Wert G, Dondorp W, et al. Recent developments in genetics and medically assisted reproduction: From research to clinical applications. European Journal of Human Genetics. 2018;**26**(1):12-33

[112] Klutstein M, Gonen N. Epigenetic aging of mammalian gametes. Molecular Reproduction and Development. 2023;**90**(12):785-803

[113] Sciorio R, Cantatore C, D'Amato G, Smith GD. Cryopreservation, cryoprotectants, and potential risk of epigenetic alteration. Journal of Assisted Reproduction and Genetics. 2024;**41**(11):2953-2967

[114] Liu XS, Wu H, Ji X, Stelzer Y, Wu X, Czauderna S, et al. Editing DNA methylation in the mammalian genome. Cell. 2016;**167**(1):233-247.e17

[115] Amabile A, Migliara A, Capasso P, Biffi M, Cittaro D, Naldini L, et al. Inheritable silencing of endogenous genes by hit-and-run targeted epigenetic editing. Cell. 2016;**167**(1):219-232.e14

[116] Osman E, Franasiak J, Scott R. Oocyte and embryo manipulation and epigenetics. Seminars in Reproductive Medicine. 2018;**36**(3-4):e1-e9

[117] Srirattana K, St John JC. Additional mitochondrial DNA influences the interactions between the nuclear and mitochondrial genomes in a bovine embryo model of nuclear transfer. Scientific Reports. 2018;**8**(1):7246

[118] Khadivi F, Razavi S, Hashemi F. Protective effects of zinc on rat sperm chromatin integrity involvement: DNA methylation, DNA fragmentation, ubiquitination and protamination after bleomycin etoposide and cis-platin treatment. Theriogenology. 2020;**142**:177-183

[119] Reyes Palomares A, Rodriguez-Wallberg KA. Update on the epigenomic implication of embryo cryopreservation methods applied in assisted reproductive technologies with potential long-term health effects. Frontiers in Cell and Development Biology. 2022;**10**:881550

[120] Mani S, Ghosh J, Coutifaris C, Sapienza C, Mainigi M. Epigenetic changes and assisted reproductive technologies. Epigenetics. 2020;**15**(1-2):12-25

[121] Yu X, Xu J, Song B, Zhu R, Liu J, Liu YF, et al. The role of epigenetics in women's reproductive health: The impact of environmental factors. Frontiers in Endocrinology. 2024;**15**:1399757

[122] Schandera J, Mackey TK. Mitochondrial replacement techniques: Divergence in global policy. Trends in Genetics. 2016;**32**(7):385-390

[123] Cohen IG, Adashi EY, Gerke S, Palacios-González C, Ravitsky V. The regulation of mitochondrial replacement techniques around the world. Annual Review of Genomics and Human Genetics. 2020;**21**:565-586